W9-CLA-679

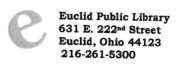

African Americans and Depression

African Americans and Depression

Signs, Awareness, Treatments, and Interventions

Julia F. Hastings, Lani V. Jones, and
Pamela P. Martin

ROWMAN & LITTLEFIELD
Lanham • Boulder • New York • London

Published by Rowman & Littlefield
A wholly owned subsidiary of The Rowman & Littlefield Publishing Group, Inc.
4501 Forbes Boulevard, Suite 200, Lanham, Maryland 20706
www.rowman.com

Unit A, Whitacre Mews, 26-34 Stannary Street, London SE11 4AB

British Library Cataloguing in Publication Information Available

Library of Congress Cataloging-in-Publication Data
Hastings, Julia F. (Julia Faye), 1969- , author.
African Americans and depression : Signs, awareness, treatments, and interventions / Julia F. Hastings, Lani V. Jones, and Pamela P. Martin.
p. cm.
Includes bibliographical references and index.
ISBN 978-1-4422-3031-6 (cloth : alk. paper) -- ISBN 978-1-4422-3032-3 (electronic)
I. Jones, Lani V. (Lani Valencia), author. II. Martin, Pamela P. (Pamela Paulette), author. III. Title.
[DNLM: 1. Depression--United States. 2. Depressive Disorder--United States. 3. African Americans--United States, 4. Community Mental Health Services--United States. 5. Health Policy--United States. WM 171.5]
RC537
616.85'27008996073--dc23
2015001363

∞ ™ The paper used in this publication meets the minimum requirements of American National Standard for Information Sciences Permanence of Paper for Printed Library Materials, ANSI/NISO Z39.48-1992.

Printed in the United States of America

Contents

Preface

Julia F. Hastings

As African Americans, we collectively wish for good health. However, what does *good health* mean when good health and seeking timely information are riddled with barriers? What complexities are introduced to living a life of *good health* when, for some African American people, there is inescapable worry about the future? What meaning does life hold when mental illness is unrecognized because the fight to keep going demands overcoming struggle? Answers to these questions are not easy.

We, the authors, write this book to offer information about one particular mental illness causing pain and devastation—clinical depression. In all its forms, depression causes many African Americans to suffer in silence because verbalizing sadness is equated with weakness in character. The strong expectation of denying every sad event continues to be a cultural norm, but the heaviness of thoughts, pains, and experiences often leads to untenable living. Given current scientific findings and social reporters, many barriers to good health for African Americans exist despite efforts to improve access to care. What can be done to shed light on this very personal condition?

A book about African Americans and depression is timely given the escalating reports of tragedy in the United States. Depression remains tied to the complex web of the greatest social challenges—poverty, discrimination, declining health as we age, community unrest, addictions, and interrupted pursuits of happiness. Learning about shootings, killings, drug overdoses, and domestic violence occurrences in our communities leaves almost no escape from feeling the weight of tragedy. Being directly affected by misfortune makes coping with some of life's events overwhelming. Seeking help from strangers—mental health professionals—compounds the difficulty to maintain optimal physical health balance and good mental health.

African Americans experience the lowest life expectancy and the highest mortality rate of all racial, ethnic, and gender groups in the United States.[1] Staggering health care inequities in all disease areas and medical services also contribute to bleak findings. When focusing on mental illness, Black Americans still face discrimination in diagnosis, facility accessibility, treatment type, length of care, and follow-up care. The medical and therapeutic disparities alone impede optimal health. Changes must be made to counter such a dismal situation. Depression is painful, isolating, and destroys lives indiscriminately.

We wish to share our knowledge, practice experiences, and research findings with those searching for a pathway to relief. Experiencing emotional lows does not mean attitude or character weakness. Being afflicted with the symptoms of depression does not mean one loses a connection with spirituality. Depression's burden impacts all of African American society from individuals to the population at large. Consequently, we believe one step in improving the mental health status of African Americans is knowledge.

This book evolved naturally over fifteen years from discussions among ourselves, the authors. Family, friends, neighbors, and colleagues around the country also inspired ideas outlining this subject matter. We quickly realized the gap between conversations on depression and its specific effects on African Americans. We rarely experienced attention to our culture and our history. Talking about depression might be viewed as a betrayal to our ancestors and, therefore, is treated as a taboo topic. Sadly, U.S. history plays a part in the pattern of blatant negligence when recognizing mental illness among African American people. Who are we to suggest weakness among a people who have survived under the harshest conditions beginning with slavery? We hope this book launches conversations outside the hushed tones of taboo. Most importantly, this work must serve to catalyze action for improved care.

African Americans and Depression is groundbreaking in that it is among the first books to be written for the general population, focusing primarily on the needs of African Americans. One pressing question is, "Why complete this book now?" To be truthful, there is never a really good time to write a book on this subject. Throughout American history the mental health status of African Americans has always been in question, and, according to Professor James S. Jackson, a noted researcher on Black mental health, has been "used to justify slavery, enforce racial segregation, and reinforce the idea that blacks were inferior to whites."[2] Historically, supporting the notion that African Americans experienced depression detracted from acknowledged personhood.

The book focuses primarily on the psychological and medical needs of African Americans. African Americans, historically and presently, have dealt with a series of inescapable burdens. Before, during, and after the Civil Rights Era, African Americans wrestled with notions of personhood, federal restrictions, "redlining" housing policies, and indescribable violence from hostile forces. Beyond dealing with everyday prejudice, communities of color were also ostracized and policed due to official laws and unofficial social practices. With such restrictions came suspicion based upon demeaning stereotypes both from popular culture and racist perceptions. Therefore, the pressures of discrimination besiege the body with high blood pressure, stress, and fear as daily life is meted out on prejudicial terms. In the mind, the constant tension from acts of racism and hostility draws the sufferer into a deeper well of depression. Sadly, because of the historical denial about mental health conditions among African Americans, messages about good mental health within a cultural schema are often difficult to sustain.

In addition to domestic issues, heartache, anger, and frustration from the less-than-polite aspects of society only produce melancholy and hopelessness. Social media delivers more unseemly, nasty commentary from anonymous individuals who openly speak their minds about their hatred for African Americans. Such rhetoric does not appear only on blogs or forums, but even on more official sources such as educational websites and newspapers. The African American persona shoulders a beating on a daily basis. It is no wonder that depression and other aspects of mental illness cause a level of inconsolability. We need to provide resources that offer a place of solace from hurt and silent despair. This book launches such an investigation in order to make sense of the chaos that African Americans experience within the deepest levels of the mind.

Sometimes, such historical, political, and attitudinal social relations transfer over into the care an African American receives from health practitioners. Unfortunately, African Americans may see therapeutic professionals as advisors who do not respect culture or race. Because of these barriers to cultural communication, one cannot truly get the help one needs. Therefore, the affected person feels lost and truly unable to express the haunting nature of depression. If the therapist implements considerate actions and respect, the African American client can learn to deal with painful issues properly. Additionally, the mental health professional will not be viewed as an enemy but, rather, as a friendly ally on the path to healing from psychological pain.

We write this book to address an overlooked issue in the African American community. There are many accounts of depression from the first-person perspective, and there are scattered resources for all to find on the Internet, but not all resources are reliable. Such available resources also include the "learned" community of professionals who do not agree on a singular message about the depression care process or treatment provisions for African Americans because many related symptoms are dismissed as being temporary. In reality, depression is treatable. While earlier treatment seeking is better, we wish for our readers to understand that it is never too late to seek help. We hope the words on the following pages instill hope, offer a sense of direction, and renew spirits about how depression can be addressed with cultural appropriateness and responsiveness.

ORGANIZATION OF THIS BOOK

The book begins with an introduction to depression among African Americans and lays the foundation for all subsequent chapters. Following the introduction to the signs of and cultural myths surrounding depression, the book contains five key areas. The first chapter defines depression and what it means for African Americans. Chapter 2 explains how to seek professional help and overcome barriers to access. The following chapter covers a variety of community interventions and innovations in service programs. Examples describe popular and effective treatment options occurring in the community. New directions in the U.S. medical and mental health care systems because of recent policy changes are addressed in chapter 4. Chapter 5 offers our parting thoughts about next steps. To facilitate further interest, we offer an appendix on popular resources available to the general public. The suggestions outlined will help you or your loved ones embark on a journey toward fulfillment and wellness. We hope the book will inspire the reader to discover that depression is not an end, but a beginning in growth and understanding.

Acknowledgments

The authors wish to acknowledge the people who have helped to make this book possible. THANK YOU to all who provided support, talked things over, read, wrote, provided comments, served as research participants, LISTENED, PRAYED, and offered unyielding FAITH that this book would see the light of day. We dedicate this book to our ancestors, families, friends, and the wise ears that have been burdened with hearing about "the book." We hope that when you read our words you find comfort, information that is helpful, feel our unwavering energy and dedication to focus on Black people, and experience a launching point to make public a very private, and sometimes culturally shameful, condition. It is our goal to chip away at the shamefulness and the tendency to ignore the cherished souls of our people.

JFH: To the Hastings family—Cecilia especially—no words can express my dependency on all you do in private to make my public life worthy of print. Your unwavering prayers, support, and encouragement to be a better person, in spite of (or because of) my many moods, are beyond what I have given in return. I am also grateful to the people I call mentors and close friends who keep me on a positive path! Your support, words of wisdom, and tangible efforts to help me on this journey never go unnoticed. You know who you are without a name drop. I will cherish your guidance and our friendship always. Lunch next week? Allow me one name—Dean Katharine Briar-Lawson; you found a way to offer me safe passage in the storm. No words can convey the depth of my appreciation for your understanding the inexplicable. I am able to live my dream of being the kind of scholar that can make a difference in many lives because of your insight, patience (ten years!), and ability to help others navigate roads less traveled.

Research reported in this book was supported by the National Institute on Minority Health and Health Disparities of the National Institutes of Health under award number 7K22MD00393402. *Disclaimer*: The content is solely the responsibility of the authors and does not necessarily represent the official views of the National Institutes of Health.

LVJ: Much of what I have learned over the years as a feminist-scholar came as the result of my work with mental health consumers, all of whom, in their own ways, inspired me and subconsciously contributed a tremendous amount to the content of this book via their stories of pain, fear, and rejection. I am grateful to have been invited into your healing circle.

I am very grateful to a number of friends (although I am unable to name you all) for their strong support and constant encouragement shown through many phone calls and/or texts. To my sister-friends, Francine Guy, Laura Colaneri, Vanessa Jackson, and Lynn A. Warner, who talked things over, read, wrote, and provided moral support throughout some challenging times—I'm deeply indebted. In honor of my grandma Ethel Mae, Mom (aka Slim), and sister Mel, who imparted the experiential seeds of "worry" but "wisdoms" of healing through storytelling, without whom the completion of this book would not have been possible—Ashe.

PPM: I want to give thanks for the many blessings of being a coauthor on this book. I personally want to thank Dr. Julia F. Hastings and Dr. Lani V. Jones. As a person who stands on her faith, I want to thank my prayer partner and friend, Dr. LaTrese Adkins. I want to thank my family and friends who shared their own personal stories about maintaining their own positive psychological well-being.

We are also grateful to our editor, Suzanne Staszak-Silva, for her kind words, feedback, guidance, and support while working on the book. Your patience, encouragement, and ability to give us time and space to write is beyond words. May this group effort launch new beginnings.

Chapter One

Understanding the Signs of Depression

Julia F. Hastings

NOT "JUST THE BLUES"

Grace. Faith. Hope. Living vibrantly. As each day passes we expect to experience joy, pain, sorrow, and utter fulfillment. Sometimes, we experience the entire spectrum of emotions in one day. As an African people, we embody our ancestors' survival instincts when living through the cruelest actions meant to break the soul. Our strength as a people has always been discovering ways to maintain personhood against many adversities. Even in the present day, we continue to use this practice as a survival instinct. Having the presence of mind to maintain composure in the face of utter hardship bestows dignity in the face of brutality. From the violence and chaos of the Reconstruction Era to the ugliness of Jim Crow, staying strong ensured protection for ourselves and for our loved ones. The fight and eventual granting of rights from the civil rights movement planted the seeds of change and growth as an emancipated community of individuals. Despite these milestones, the mere indignities of racism and societal stigma did not go away. Institutional discrimination from an unforgiving society still stung. As a community, the denial of city services, the failing school systems, and vicious neighborhood violence are roadblocks in our fight to remain whole.

Our elders and parents often quipped that difficult times create stronger people. Because of what African Americans endured since touching the soil of the New World in the seventeenth century, maintaining strength became the cornerstone of thriving in the face of insurmountable odds. However, this cultural belief unleashes new and profound questions when dealing with the effects of suffering as a societal outgroup. Does this cultural belief based on hurt, rejection, and the continued sadness of our history in this society solely depict "just the blues"? Is the impact of the blues based on how the outer society reacts to us as a whole? How does "being blue" resonate with us as individuals? Accepting chaos as a normal behavioral process produces a caustic lifestyle in which denial becomes more apparent than self-fulfillment. Joy becomes replaced by frustration and anger. Ultimately, one feels lost and buried under feeling dejected and apathetic in the face of tough odds.

Endurance over hardship transforms into a "triumph over adversity" mentality that has been passed down from each generation to the next. Such a mentality entails much effort, personal fortitude, and resilience. Reclaiming the courage to challenge adverse forces means reassessing personal worth. Feeling helpless in the face of such cultural beliefs requires a different sort of courage. Instead of trying to "remain strong" and continuing to suffer, reclaiming the courage to request aid is necessary in order to function in society. Overwhelming pressures eventually break down the wall of strength and send forth a wave of pent-up pain that only has scratched the surface.

As a community, the belief in optimism despite the choices we make supports character. Feeling hopeful in times of utter despair becomes a coping mechanism that keeps us whole when everything else seems not to work. At the same time, simply remaining positive also throws a cover over the truth behind the pain. Hiding behind a façade only drags the sufferer deeper into the quagmire of self-doubt and denial. The mask of hiding one's troubles from the world becomes more solidified. Depression can be experienced mentally and physically, and the sadness that characterizes it does not go away on its own. Faith alone does not bring solace. In the end, the inability to find meaning within the confines of religion leads to what is called "experiencing the blues."

Among the lives of many African Americans, the "blues" is no stranger. Our art, words, and songs reflect bouts of sadness. An entire genre of music grew out of vocalizing pain. Authors such as James Baldwin and Richard Wright painted ugly scenarios built from the ache of facing racism. Nevertheless, art slowly morphed into real experience for everyday people. Living circumstances, especially in American society, produce an understanding of quiet struggle and long endurance while facing hard times. Additionally, our culture subscribes to the tolerance of the most volatile discrimination and anger from individuals and societal institutions. With this daily assault on self-respect, the right to exist truly becomes an ordeal. Our presence, life purpose, and goals are derided by a consistent lack of cultural understanding.

There is no single cause of depression, as has been identified by science. Scientific research has established that a combination of genetic, biological, environmental, and psychological factors stand as root causes. Many African Americans with depression-like symptoms never seek treatment. For some who ask the question, "Why me, Lord?" one of the first places to seek assistance is religion. Turning to the church for guidance provides a salve for the wounds inflicted by the outside world. Bible teachings reaffirm our faith in humankind. Reading scripture undergirds our intention to exist. The mind-body connection reflects no separateness in our culture when based on faith.

When one suffers with depression, carrying out daily activities creates an intense tug-of-war between low times and ease. Sleeping becomes a necessary refuge. Being awake resembles torturous action. Eating more than our average meal leads to feeling guilty about the act of indulgence in the face of moderation. Bouts of overeating change into tremendous guilt about weight gain. Experiencing endless isolation overtakes anything else in the depth of despondency and lack of self-worth. The actions and emotions during such melancholy collectively contribute to life's lowest point.

Such behavioral and psychological events weave themselves into a state of melancholy. Sadly, this melancholy can be intensified by the contradictions created by its own symptoms. For example, hiding away from the world can cause sufferers of depression to feel an even deeper loss and feelings of isolation and hurt, and yet human contact becomes a chore rather than a pleasure. Similarly, the happiness and fulfillment of certain activities lose their luster. Once joyous hobbies now seem boring and drab. Going to sleep is now a battle of wills. Insomnia takes over, and rest develops into an endless chore. One thing is certain: depression may be at the center of mood swings. Yet the question still remains whether we can tell the difference between a "bad patch" and something more serious. After all, African Americans generationally learned to remain strong and deny pain. Feelings of depression dwell in secrecy and silence.

This depth of loneliness carves an emotional scar that continues to make its presence known as the days pass. African Americans continue to silently endure despite the emotional wrestling that is a result of depression. Unfortunately, not being able to vocalize the deep pain psychically and physically contributes to an even deeper wound from harsh experiences. In this chapter, we learn about defining depression culturally, what signs of depression to be aware of, and how a diagnosis might be provided. The chapter also offers a discussion on how many African American people suffer from depression by gender and age. Concluding this chapter is an overview of how emergency rooms and emergency psychiatric services might serve as launching points for intervention.

AFRICAN AMERICAN CULTURE AND DEPRESSION

Many African Americans underestimate the impact of mental illness, and depression in particular, on daily functioning. African American culture in the United States is distinct, as it is rooted in African practices or behaviors, customs, and food. Developing over time, African American culture represents a combination of values and beliefs that honors ancestors, outlines separate roles for men and women, incorporates religiosity and spirituality, and establishes coping strategies for life events. Roughly forty-two million people identify as African American according to the 2013 U.S. Census Bureau.[1] Twenty-five percent of this population earned incomes below the poverty level.[2]

Many aspects of culture offer protection from harm and function as a foundation for resilience. Other cultural aspects might lead to declines in health. Distinct traditions developed over time to nurture the African American spirit such as song, oral history narratives, ancestor remembrances, and worship. Using culture allows African Americans to eliminate or modify problems, reframe the meaning of events or situations, and manage the level of emotional response.[3]

A common cultural behavior involves toiling through tough situations using high effort. However, this relentless behavior produces wear and tear on the human body such that poor health may result in forms of depression and high blood pressure. Researchers connect eventual poor health outcomes of African Americans to *John Henryism*.[4] The life of a hard worker might resemble the legendary West Virginian John Henry, a famous freedman steelworker who gave his life for a construction contest. John Henryism defines a strong behavioral predisposition to cope actively with environmental stressors. In other words, working to exhaustion with little reward.

Developed by public health researcher Sherman James, John Henryism represents the ability to continue working without ever voicing concern until one literally breaks down.[5] African American men and women constantly endure exceedingly perilous social interactions and events until harm lethally strikes health later in the life course. Disturbingly, being able to endure even the slightest inconvenience without complaint adds to an already heavy burden of bad health with poor health care connections. Sadly for the character of the well-loved story, John Henry dies of exhaustion after succeeding in his challenge. Behind his martyrdom lies another epiphany: his selfless act had put forth a dangerous perception of the ideal national acculturation adaptation for African Americans. For an African American to be accepted and even "acknowledged" within the fabric of the United States, he or she must be able to suffer in silence. Acceptance of larger ideals adds to the detriment of health, sanity, and character. In the end, an individual might be praised, but at what cost?

Despite the cultural value of staying focused during tough and unwieldy times, depression still represents a formidable challenge. Everyone concerned with African American mental health must focus on depression and its underestimated impact on well-being. In fact, depression's grasp on daily functioning is so treacherous that it affects the economic and social fate of individuals and communities. Sometimes, possessing a strong will is not enough to conquer the ravages of low socioeconomic status, low emotions, and painfully languid movement.

In the present day, stressors for African Americans quadruple. Not only do financial issues have to be dealt with, experiencing disparities in societal institutions also makes an indelibly sordid impact as well. Constant existential attacks start the drama. Thus, managing the negativity of racialized perception weighs an individual of color down. To deal with such ugliness, cultural coping skills are developed to fight against the terseness from the outside world. To the African American community, this shows utter potency against the harshness of society. Unfortunately, withstanding a lifetime of hatred, pain, and attack eats away balance and medical wellness. Being strong and resilient erodes health issues and results in the sufferer being sidelined with devastating ailments.

Stoic resilience, in itself, can be an important trait to have. In the realm of medicine, the African American patient unfortunately implements this behavior to remain mute during a physical or mental exam. Not discussing such issues with medical practitioners corresponds with the cultural norms of the African American community. The years of ill treatment from social institutions within the United States resulted in distrust and suspiciousness of those in authoritative positions. Countless stories of abuse from racial violence and strict nationwide legislation fostered anger from the community of color at large. Frequent injury to African Americans with such blatant disregard contributed to building a psychological wall of resistance. Reluctant responses eventually corresponded with the weight of depression—especially after a physician's disclosure of serious diagnoses.

One plausible explanation for the African American community to dismiss the impact of depression on daily living is the near unlikelihood of discussing symptoms with their physicians. Reluctance to share current problems is partly a result of medical mistrust, stigma, and cultural beliefs around responding to depression with stoicism. As noted by researcher David R. Williams, African Americans who perceive discrimination in health care environments are less likely to seek treatment despite the presence of multiple symptoms that detract from living peacefully.[6,7] Evidence also shows that African Americans who are treated by psychiatrists or psychologists are more likely to receive adequate depression treatment relative to those treated by primary care physicians, but that the prescribed antidepressants are less likely to be taken as directed.[8] Thus, the low rate of care by mental health specialists may contribute to the widely publicized low rates of guideline-concordant care prescribed.

Another aspect of African American culture arises with the connection to church/spirituality. The church provides membership into a community, a safe haven, and a place to feel emotionally connected. The church is also a place to connect mind, body, and spirit. "Being spiritual" means supporting the belief that the human soul is connected to something separate from our place on earth. It also means believing in forgiveness—of ourselves and of others. Prayer is powerful.

Religious commitment is high among many African Americans. For some who admit to not regularly attending church services, many still readily admit to "growing up in" the church.[9] Prayer and reading Bible passages rank among the most common ways of coping with stress, illness, and difficult times. Holding on to "faith" that God will show you the way is frequently upheld as a characteristic of being strong. Attitudes about faith include believing that the current situation is only temporary and that asking other people for help and assistance with depressed feelings is only a sign of weakness. The truth is, individuals gain strength from beginning the helping process.

"TAKING MY TROUBLES TO JESUS" (DEPRESSION MYTHS)

The intersection between African Americans, culture, spirituality, and depression sometimes creates barriers to seeking treatment, perpetuates misinformation and confusion, and, unfortunately, expands the cultural myths shrouded around mental illness in the community. Myths about depression can keep people from getting proper treatment. The following statements reflect some common misconceptions about African Americans and depression (excerpts from Terrie M. Williams's 2009 book)[10]:

- "Why are you depressed? If our people could make it through slavery, we can make it through anything."
- "When a Black woman suffers from a mental disorder, the opinion is that she is weak. And weakness in Black women is intolerable."
- "You should take your troubles to Jesus, not some stranger/psychiatrist."

Spiritual support can be an important part of healing, but the care of a qualified mental health professional is essential. The earlier treatment begins, the more effective it can be.

DEPRESSION: DIAGNOSIS, SIGNS, AND SYMPTOMS

The question as to whether African Americans, and Black people overall, exhibit different behavioral cues of depression remains debatable. To understand African American expressions, one first might look at the signs found on the Internet, in textbooks, and commonly taught in university courses on mental illness. The first onset of depression may occur at any time. Many African Americans may experience a single episode of depression following a one time stressful event and recover without any future experiences. Others who experience one episode will experience symptoms that may not reach diagnosis level but cause increased impairment. Others experience impaired functioning at work and/or are unable to maintain friendships, familial relationships, or marital roles. It is more important to understand the age of onset. People who are diagnosed with depression at younger ages may experience worse symptoms, and the length between episodes might shorten with time. The course of depression is different for each person and, therefore, the chance for recurrence, severe impairment, and chronicity will differ as well. Most diagnosed depressions first appear in the teenage years and early twenties (adulthood).[11,12]

Clinical depression is not something that a friend or family member can assess. However, family and friends are probably the first to acknowledge the signs that "something" is different about a person. Family members should pay attention to key signs, such as declines in academic advancement in school, poor planning for employment, distance from social connections, and increasing participation in risky, stressful situations. All members of the family are affected, and those with symptoms of depression tend to draw attention to and largely focus on negative circumstances.

Health care professionals and insurance companies use the *Diagnostic and Statistical Manual of Mental Disorders*,[13] fifth edition (DSM-V) to document the presence of mental conditions. In the United States and much of the world, the DSM-V is considered the best handbook for clinicians to follow in order to make a diagnosis. The DSM-V contains descriptions, symptoms, and other criteria for diagnosing mental conditions. Each category of mental illness provides a common language for communication about symptom clusters and helps to establish consistent diagnoses that can also be reinterpreted by researchers. For more information about the DSM-V, see http://www.dsm5.org/about/Pages/Default.aspx. Experiencing five or more symptoms for longer than two weeks, feeling suicidal, or believing that experienced symptoms interfere with daily routine all serve as signs to seek the opinion of a medical or mental health professional. The following list of symptoms is generally accepted as commonly reported when clinical depression might be considered as a diagnosis.

Excerpt of Symptoms Used in Diagnosing Clinical Depression

- A persistent sad, anxious, or "empty" mood, or excessive crying
- Reduced appetite and weight loss or increased appetite and weight gain
- Persistent physical symptoms that do not respond to treatment, such as headaches, digestive disorders, and chronic pain
- Irritability, restlessness
- Decreased energy, fatigue, feeling "slowed down"

- Feelings of guilt, worthlessness, helplessness, hopelessness, pessimism
- Sleeping too much or too little, early-morning waking
- Loss of interest or pleasure in activities, including sex
- Difficulty concentrating, remembering, or making decisions
- Thoughts of death or suicide, or suicide attempts

In Dr. Julia Hastings's recent study, "Understanding Diabetes and Depression among African Americans in California and New York,"[14] participants shared a variety of reactions to receiving a clinical diagnosis. Some were relieved, others felt more sadness, and yet a few reported initiating treatment. All told, the reactions shared below represent only a few examples of the many emotions experienced after receiving a clinical depression diagnosis:

- I was shocked because I never thought I'd ever have any type of mental problem that would affect my life.
- I was not surprised because depression runs in my family.
- I started to get depressed after my doctor's visit. I've been depressed probably for six months but I'm getting better because I got help.
- I felt relief. Someone finally understood me.
- My first reaction was sadness. Now what am I gonna do?
- I started talking. Saying everything that I felt. I said I constantly get headaches. My back is in constant pain. I haven't been able to get proper care, I believe.
- I felt relief then I would say hopeless because it's just one more thing in my life to deal with.
- I thought, "Thank God!" I am finally going to get better!
- I started crying and couldn't stop.
- Oh, I wasn't diagnosed as a child. My mother always knew something was a little bit wrong with me. . . . She just knew something was going on with me, because she could just see this mania and stuff and I had these mood swings and stuff like that. When I was diagnosed, I was so sad because I got fired off of that job and had that CNA license and I didn't think I'd get another job. Later on down the line, fast-forward it, I got really sick on meth and stuff and that's when my mental health went really down, really bad. . . . After my diagnosis, I am happy I was placed in the hospital. The hospital put me on a good path. Thinking back, I've come a long way, but I needed help.

WHO DOES DEPRESSION AFFECT? (EPIDEMIOLOGY)

Major depression is a common and disabling psychiatric disorder. World-wide, it is the fourth leading cause of disability and the leading cause of nonfatal disease burden, accounting for almost 12 percent of total years lived with disability.[15] Major depression affects Whites (17.9 percent) at a higher lifetime rate than for African Americans (10.4 percent).[16] African American women experience major depression (12 percent) two times more than men (6 percent), and according to Dr. David R. Williams and his research team, African Americans who are employed experience major depression at lower rates than unemployed African Americans.[17]

Life Expectancy and African Americans with Depression

Life expectancy at birth has historically been shorter for African Americans than other Americans, but the large differences shorten at older ages for women (table 1.1). According to the Centers for Disease Control and Prevention, African American life expectancy, on average, is three years less than for non-Hispanic White Americans, but Blacks are also far less likely to self-report major depression. Experiencing depression may shorten longevity among African Americans due to longer durations between the acknowledgment of symptoms and treatment seeking. As of 2013, African American women in the United States had a life expectancy at birth of 78.0 years, and African American men 71.8 years.[18] However, at age 75, life expectancy for African American women is 12.5 additional years and 10.2 years for African American men. This increase in longevity is partly due to advancements in medical technology and improving prescription drug treatment adherence, as well as better access to care due to attention to the disparities in health research literature that began with the recognized differences in treatment reported in the Institute of Medicine's 2002 report.[19]

How Do African American Women Experience Depression?

African American women are recognized as the most undertreated group for depression in the United States.[20] It is becoming increasingly clear that poverty, single parenting, goal-striving stress, and racial and gender discrimination place African American women at greater risk for depression. Women are more likely to attempt suicide compared to men. Finally, approximately 10 to 15 percent of African American women experience postpartum depression (depression after childbirth) the first few weeks after delivery.[21] Symptoms of postpartum depression include crying, anxiety, insomnia, poor appetite, irritability, and lack of interest in her new baby. These symptoms may cause new mothers to feel isolated, guilty, or ashamed and can be difficult to

Table 1.1. Life Expectancy by Age Group and Race, in Years, 2013

Life Expectancy	Total Population— All Races	White	African American		
	Both Sexes	Both Sexes	Both Sexes	Men	Women
At Birth	78.7	78.9	75.1	71.8	78.0
At Age 65 (additional years)	19.1	19.2	17.8	15.9	19.3
At Age 75 (additional years)	12.1	12.1	11.6	10.2	12.5

Source: U.S. Department of Health and Human Services, Centers for Disease Control and Prevention, National Center for Health Statistics, "Health, United States, 2013: With Special Feature on Prescription Drugs."

distinguish from depression. Usually, the postpartum depression symptoms go away in about three weeks.

Women may be more likely to display emotional responses related to depression including sadness, feeling empty, showing difficulty in making decisions, expressing feelings of guilt or worthlessness, and entertaining thoughts of death and suicide. African American women may delay seeking help for depression by being more prone to ignoring emotional responses and seeking comfort from religion. Religious coping may be associated with maladaptive or avoidant coping strategies for African American women because comfort may be experienced.[22] Participating in religious activities may serve as a survival activity as well.

How Do African American Men Experience Depression?

Men are more likely to report being very tired, exhibit irritability, lose interest in once pleasurable activities, and have difficulty sleeping. In general, these signs suggest that men are less likely to report feelings of sadness, worthlessness, and even excessive guilt.[23]

Men may be more likely than women to turn to alcohol or drugs when they are depressed. Some men also may become frustrated, discouraged, irritable, angry, sometimes abusive toward others, and/or behave recklessly. Although more women may attempt suicide, a higher number of men die by violent suicide in the United States.[24]

How Do African American Children and Adolescents Experience Depression?

African American children and adolescents who develop depression often have more severe and frequent episodes in adulthood.[25] Signs a child may be experiencing depression may include pretending to be sick, refusing to go to school, acting clingy to a parent, or excessively worrying that a parent may die. Older children may sulk, get into trouble at school, be negative and irritable, and feel misunderstood. It may be difficult to accurately diagnose a young person with depression because these signs may resemble normal, developmentally appropriate mood swings.[26]

How Do Older African American Adults Experience Depression?

When older African American adults experience depression, it may be over-looked because seniors may show different, less obvious symptoms. Some-times depression can be difficult to distinguish from grief. After the loss of a loved one, grief represents a normal reaction to the loss and generally does not require professional mental health treatment. However, grief that is complicated and lasts for a very long time following a loss may require treatment. Depression is not a normal part of aging, and older adults may be less likely to admit to feelings of sadness or grief. Since older adults experience more medical conditions such as heart disease, stroke, or cancer, caregivers need to be more diligent about potential depressive symptoms. The same caution should be followed if older adults are taking medications with side effects.

Landmark reports in 2001 by the former surgeon general of the United States, Dr. David Satcher[27] and in 2003 by the Institute of Medicine[28] called attention to the ethnic minority population's limited access to high-quality health and mental health care. Reviewers indicated that African Americans appear not to suffer from higher levels of mental illness than Whites.[29] There are methodological reasons to question the legitimacy of this counterintuitive finding.[30] Consensus is strong, however, that mentally ill African Americans receive less outpatient treatment than Whites from social workers and other trained professionals who provide specialty mental health treatment.[31,32] At community and societal levels, depression is a costly condition. Costs associated with depression, including those for direct care (inpatient, outpatient, and pharmaceutical), suicide-related events, and workplace burdens (i.e., absenteeism and reduced productivity), rose from $52.9 billion in 1990 to $83.1 billion in 2000 and in 2013, over $118 billion.[33,34] Because of treatment access disparities exacerbated by wide differences in the quality of care,[35] untreated depression and other untreated mental illnesses impose a disproportionate disease burden on African American communities.[36]

Untreated mental illness imposes considerable psychological distress, and for that reason alone, professionals and researchers should figure out how to reduce the likelihood of undiagnosed cases. Less widely acknowledged is how much untreated mental illness compromises the mentally ill person's ability to meet day-to-day responsibilities and the person's ability to function as a productive member of his or her family and community. More than half of people suffering from depression cannot function well in meeting social obligations as a result of their mental illness.[37]

ECONOMY AND COMMUNITY

Understanding the impact of poverty remains important to learning about depression among African Americans. Poverty affects not only individuals and families, but also communities and society. Living in rural or urban areas makes little difference within the African American populations because each location tends to contain concentrated poverty where social problems accumulate. Many impoverished areas suffer from few resources, extreme building distress, high unemployment rates, homelessness, high residential turnover, substance abuse, and increasing crime.[38] Neighborhood and community problems impede generalized trust among neighbors, erode mechanisms of resistance to social control (i.e., voting power, protesting, etc.), and can decrease individual mental functioning that may lead to episodes of depression.

The economic social context also affects African Americans with depression because of the larger impacts on the economy. Although the U.S. economy varies from region to region, research has consistently shown that African Americans remain especially vulnerable to longer unemployment spells than other racial counterparts, accumulate little wealth, and are many times directly affected by cyclical downturns in the economy.[39,40] Maintaining the economic well-being of African Americans also must be understood within context. It is important to consider the impact of the economy on depression within African Americans because access (insurance status), treatment choices, social support, and condition improvement are all tied together. It is likely that the social and material resources needed to make inroads in improving mental states are at the center of where the focus will be targeted on improving quality, culturally focused interventions.

AFRICAN AMERICANS AND EMERGENCY MEDICAL AND PSYCHIATRIC EMERGENCY SERVICES

The emergency medical services system has grown and has become increasingly complex. As reported by the Institute of Medicine in a 2007 report on emergency medical services, emergency departments received almost 114 million visits, most often for chest pain, shortness of breath, stomach pain, and injury from many causes including motor vehicle accidents.[41] The economically disadvantaged and the uninsured most particularly rely extensively on emergency medical services. For many emergency medical services users, its constant availability—even with long waiting periods—leads to it serving as a frequent source of health care.

African Americans are overrepresented among emergency medical services users—the African American emergency department visit rate is about twice the White rate.[42] Because of poverty,[43] physical illness, and other vulnerabilities that are risk factors for mental illness, emergency medical services users are at a greater risk for mental illness.

Nevertheless, rates of mental illness and mental health referral among emergency services users have not yet been reliably ascertained. We do know that diagnosed mental illness among emergency services users is unrealistically low and that diagnosed rates are especially low among African Americans.[44] Because data are lacking on meaningful approximations about emergency room visits for access to mental health services, African Americans experience the gate keeping process which hinders immediate care. It is beyond our capacity to calculate the amount of service provision for mental health care. Nevertheless, in view of African Americans' overrepresentation in emergency department services and what promise to be high rates of mental illness, it is reasonable to believe that emergency departments do play, or could play, a significant role in brokering mental health treatment.

Psychiatric emergency services operate as a separate system in many locales, partially due to the special nature of mental health crises. Unlike medical emergencies, mental health crises sometimes can pose a public safety concern. Persons in psychiatric crisis sometimes represent a danger to themselves or others, and can be involuntarily detained for that reason. Emergency services function as a triage point for clinical evaluation of grave disability or whether the person poses a danger to himself or herself or to others or represents one criterion for involuntary psychiatric confinement. African Americans are more likely to be considered gravely disabled or a danger to themselves or others and to be subject to involuntary commitment.[45,46] Whether or not emergency intervention results in involuntary detention, psychiatric emergency service personnel deliver a kind of mental health treatment and often make referrals for continuing care.

Surprisingly few data are available, but they indicate that African Americans are overrepresented among psychiatric emergency services.

SUMMARY

It is clear from this chapter that connecting African American historical roots with contemporary social experiences calls for more focused attention. Depression is a commonly occurring, seriously impairing, and an underdiagnosed illness for African Americans. The research evidence suggests that depression usually occurs in the twenties, but can occur more frequently as African Americans age. An essential component in improving diagnosis and therapeutic intervention is continued efforts to understand the mechanisms underlying depression. Researchers and professional clinicians need to take into account the complex society African Americans live in and especially pay attention to consumer literacy about the illness, social supports—both positive and negative—and the role of culture. Everyday events can lead to impairments that, in turn, lead to poorer performance in self-maintenance, work activities, and social roles. Researchers and clinicians also need to understand the role of insurance parity for mental health conditions and push for expanded investments in treatment options for public insurance programs. Effective treatment is dependent upon and expanded knowledge is based upon what makes African Americans similar and different over the course of depression.

Chapter Two

Permission to Heal

Lani V. Jones

Many people have a difficult time talking about depression, let alone asking for help. In fact, every year more than sixteen million Americans suffer from some type of depressive disorder.[1] The good news is that, once identified, depression can be successfully treated. And unlike in the past, when being diagnosed with a mental health disorder meant being labeled as incompetent or "crazy" forever, today people can recover and return to a normal life. Good mental health, absent of depression, helps you enjoy life and cope with problems in a healthy manner. Just as you work to take care of your body by scheduling yearly checkups with your doctors, you can do things to help protect your mental health.

Being able to recognize and talk honestly about your mental health is the first step. Sometimes it is easier to talk to a doctor, a family member, or a friend when we are sick or hurt physically, but we might prefer to keep mental health problems a secret. It isn't difficult to understand why. Shame and stigma associated with mental illness keeps us silent. You might think mental illness is something to be ashamed or afraid of. These feelings may cause you to not talk about it, especially outside of your family. As shared by a consumer, "When they (physical therapists) told me I had to go to the psych, I was so embarrassed to, I was extremely embarrassed when they told me. I was scared. I was embarrassed to tell people—my family, that I had to go to the psychiatrist, I was extremely embarrassed and didn't know what they would think about me. I did and they were more supportive than I thought."

Talking with others about your mental health struggles can help you feel better. Unfortunately, the common view that depression is a personal weakness rather than a health problem dismisses the heavy burden of the illness. This negative perception of help-seeking, often known as stigma, must be eliminated if African Americans as a community are going to help persons who live with depression to heal—*emotionally*, *physically*, and *spiritually*.[2] As shared by a consumer during a focus group, "So, it would help more to reach out to those who are struggling with depression, and have a little compassion about it. Don't put labels on them, you know. Everybody's got a label. 'Oh, she crazy (while motioning her finger),' 'He acting just like a crack-head. Oh that's an addict,' You know what I'm saying? Or 'She's on welfare. You know,' or 'She ain't never going to be nobody.' We got to stop that. Stop labeling people with mental illness and people got to stop accepting labels too."[3] If we aren't able to take care of ourselves, our families, our communities, and find ways to cope in a healthy manner, many of these negative messages are internalized without us being aware of it, causing damage to our spirits.[4]

Beyond stigma that resides in the African American community, several factors that may contribute to fewer African Americans being properly diagnosed and treated for mental health difficulties include:

- A mistrust of medical health professionals, based in part on historical higher-than-average institutionalization for African Americans with mental illness.
- Cultural barriers, influenced by language and values in the relationship between the doctor and the patient.
- Reliance on the support of family and the religious community, rather than mental health professionals, during periods of emotional distress.
- A "masking" of depressive symptoms by other medical conditions, somatic complaints, substance abuse, and other psychiatric illnesses.
- Socioeconomic factors, such as limited access to health insurance that covers mental health.

While most people experience periods when they feel sad and blue—for example, when you or a loved one is sick, going through a divorce, or having financial problems—these stressful times come and go. Your normal response may be to feel sad, frustrated, and even angry, but these are just normal responses. However, depression is beyond the feeling of having a bad day where you may feel unmotivated, disorganized, or sad. To effectively diagnose and treat depression, a licensed provider must hear about specific symptoms of depression that are occurring over a period of time, which may signify the diagnosis of clinical depression. For instance, clinical depression may cause a person either to sleep or eat to excess, or, on the contrary, to almost eliminate those activities.[5] Observable or behavioral symptoms of clinical depression also may sometimes be minimal despite a person experiencing profound inner turmoil. Depression can be an extensive disorder, and it affects a person's body, feelings, thoughts, and behaviors in a variety of ways.[6] What we are most concerned about here is when we often ignore the signs and symptoms that clearly meet the standard for depression. It is not okay for sadness or the blues to never go away. Depression is not a normal part of life for anyone. However, one's racial and/or cultural background plays a large role in how the symptoms of depression are reported and interpreted, and consequently, if and how depression is recognized and treated.[7] In particular, African Americans carry a heavy burden when it comes to depression because they are less likely than White Americans to seek mental health services or to receive proper treatment.[8] In the African American community there's a tendency to hide or ignore symptoms of depression.

Symptoms and signs of depression can range from mental and emotional to physical symptoms. They may include:

- Feeling sad or "blue"
- Confused thinking
- Withdrawal from friends and activities
- Difficulty sleeping
- Inability to cope with daily problems or stress
- Alcohol or drug abuse
- Significant changes in eating habits
- Changes in sex drive
- Excessive anger, hostility, or violence
- Suicidal thinking
- Dry mouth
- Weight gain or weight loss

Dr. Gail Wyatt says, "If we work every day and we dress well, then it's very difficult for people who don't know African Americans to see distress because it isn't always visible, but if you're disheveled and you can't get out of bed, that's easier to see."[9] As stated by a participant during a focus group meeting, "I think Black women are stronger when it comes to mental health. Oh no, we don't get close to being depressed. And we do, I think we fight it faster. I think a white person would sink in and believe it. Like a Black woman would be like 'nah, this can't be, nah.'"[10] In order to fulfill the role of the strong Black woman, many participants discussed their symptoms as being "just the blues" and downplayed the severity of their symptoms.

Historically, African Americans have normalized their own suffering. As African Americans we have been a part of historic environmental and physical traumas (cultural genocide, psychological traumas, institutional inequalities—including the health care system), which have made it necessary for us to disguise mental health issues.[11] For instance, during slavery, mental illness often resulted in a more inhumane lifestyle, including frequent beatings and abuse, which forced many slaves to hide their issues. Over time, strength became equal to survival, and showing weakness meant one might not survive. In an effort to survive, many African Americans wore the mask of survival. Paul Laurence Dunbar, in his poem "We Wear the Mask," gives eloquent witness to how African Americans had to create a structure of dissimulation in regard to their emotions tied to their daily lives as slaves and sharecroppers. But behind all that seeming is just a bunch of lies trying to cover up the fact that they were feeling pretty rotten and unable to talk about their feelings in an honest way. "We wear the mask that grins and lies, . . . With torn and bleeding hearts we smile, And mouth with myriad subtleties; Nay, let them only see us, while, we wear the mask," was first published in *Lyrics of Lowly Life* (1896) by Paul Laurence Dunbar.[12] When Dunbar writes, "With torn and bleeding hearts we smile," it is an obvious representation of the suffering felt and of how a smile is sometimes worn in order to camouflage one's true emotions.

Survival through the masking or hiding behind false appearances of wellness still exists today. Even in the workplace, African Americans continue to experience a sense of powerlessness and injustice due to discriminatory practices. One option involves masking what one may be feeling in an effort to remain employed to protect one's J-O-B and sense of pride. Enduring this daily persecution forces many African Americans to draw on their inner strength and keep silent about one's own suffering,[13] while internally, one's soul cries out with emotional pain and agony. This tendency to hide any signs or symptoms of depression means missed opportunities to intervene early with effective treatments. A part of healing includes our ability to acknowledge ourselves as emotional beings that have been and are wounded by this generational historic impact.

While history and data demonstrate that African Americans are disproportionately more likely to experience circumstances that increase their chances of having a depressive disorder, it pleads the question: Why do so many African Americans suffer in silence? How does one share their struggles with depression when they have convinced the world that they are strong? To answer these questions, we will need to be real about the ways in which African Americans have traditionally dealt with depression. This includes fighting through difficulties in isolation, being afraid and ashamed to ask for help, neglecting our own needs while taking care of others, hiding behind our pain, and dismissing the role that professional treatment can play. African Americans must come to terms with their powerlessness over depression and accept it as a temporary illness of the mind and body in order to experience an optimal level of mental health.

Seeing a mental health professional to confide in can mean the difference between illness and wellness.[14] In this chapter, we will begin our journey of mental wellness and healing. We'll talk about how to identify when we need help, how to choose a provider, potential barriers to getting the help we need, and culturally specific treatment options for depression. We'll take a close look at what we need to do to restore and preserve our mental health—and we'll help you answer the question, "Are you ready to be well?"[15]

HOW DO I KNOW IF I NEED PROFESSIONAL HELP?

Some days are harder than others. Many people experience temporary emotional ups and downs—it's a part of life. In fact, there are several personal circumstances and daily life experiences that can interfere with a balanced sense of mental wellness.[16] To name a few, everyday experiences of sexism, racism, and classism; daily work pressures; medications; physical pain and illnesses; and changes in the environment all can affect our daily mental health. Such shifts can alter our thoughts, feelings, and moods and disrupt our ability to function and relate to others.[17] To complicate matters, in many cases there's no easy way to tell when we cross over the line between going through a difficult time and actually having a depressive disorder. If you find that you're having some rough times, here are a few suggestions to get you through the day.

Try taking some time away from your normal, daily-life activities. If you can, it's good to take a mental health day from work or family or friends. Use this time or any time to take a walk around the block; to find a quiet spot in the home or outside the home to sit and reflect; to write your thoughts in a journal. Try to refocus your thoughts on the things that are going well, even if they are small. Ask yourself, "If I had a magic wand, what would I like to see different for myself?" and, "What would be my first step toward making my life different?" We can often control the negative ideas or thoughts that hold us back from having our best possible life.

If you suspect you're depressed, don't wait until you are at your lowest point: make an appointment with your medical provider and let those close to you know how you're feeling. Sometimes it's not easy to get through the rough time; you just don't have the energy or focus. For example, you may wake up one morning feeling that you got up on the wrong side of the bed and your day seems to go downhill from there. You don't have a chance to have your coffee before going out the door, and you forget your child's lunch on the kitchen counter and have to give her or him money you don't have to spare. To make matters worse, you are thirty minutes late and forgot you had a meeting at 9 a.m. However, at lunch you decide to call a friend and take a walk during the call. When you get back to your office, you feel as if you have brought it down a notch. But what happens when you don't just wake up on "the wrong side of the bed"? What if, in actuality, you do not get much sleep, and you have a hard time getting out of bed for a week. You have no energy to make lunch for your child, and you forget to make arrangements for her or him. After arriving late, you walk into the meeting disheveled and unorganized. At lunchtime your coworker recommends that you take a walk and eat something, but the best you can do is to lay your head on your desk. If these rough times persist, and you start having uncomfortable feelings or you feel as if your problems are bigger than a walk or conversation here and there, you may want to reach out for professional help.

We must be honest with ourselves about how, and what, we are feeling and look to our strengths toward addressing our mental health challenges. If we keep pretending that we're doing well, how can we ever get the help we need to live a better life? African Americans are deeply engaged in the process of caring for everyone else, which causes us to lose sight of the fact that we need nurturing ourselves. For the most part, we wait far too long to ask for help. Usually, we will only go to see a mental health care provider if our child is in trouble at school, if we experience the death of a close relative, or if we are on the verge of losing our job. It is not supposed to be that way! When something keeps you up at night, or when you become a shopaholic to make yourself feel good, or when you don't want to go to work, these are good indications that you need to talk with a professional to sort out life's happenings.

Always see your medical provider to determine whether your depression may be caused by a medical problem such as a reaction to current medications, heart problems, high blood sugar, low-grade infection, or chronic headaches. *ALERT!* If you feel suicidal or feel in danger of harming yourself or someone else, go to your nearest hospital emergency room *now*. Seeing a mental health professional to confide in and ask direction from can mean the difference between life and death. The sooner you seek help, the sooner the treatment will ease your pain, improve your quality of life, and prevent the condition from becoming worse.

WHERE CAN I GO TO GET HELP?
(ACCESS, UTILIZATION, AND NEED)

Despite national, state, and local media campaigns focused on the role of culturally specific issues in mental health care, the needs of African Americans remain marginalized.[18] What we know from research is that only one-third of African Americans with mental health difficulties use professional services. African Americans at risk of depression are less likely than their White American counterparts to have ever received mental health services and to be currently in treatment.[19] In addition, African Americans are more likely to use emergency services or to seek treatment from a primary care provider than from a mental health specialist. While hospital emergency rooms are important to many African Americans, this *should not* be the first point of access for care.[20] With a few exceptions, the field of mental health research and practice has not done a good job at understanding, naming, or effectively treating what's ailing African Americans. The President's New Freedom Commission on Mental Health (2003) described in detail the racial and cultural problems associated with service, access, and utilization in mental health, concluding that the higher burden of disability among African Americans may be attributed to treatment barriers.[21] There have been several barriers identified that African Americans face in gaining access to and using culturally responsive services: cultural barriers, cultural mistrust of medical providers, reliance on religious entities, and the lack of economic resources.[22] Specifically, this explains the interactions of race, gender, and class and how they impact wellness in a unique way among African Americans.

POTENTIAL BARRIERS FOR GETTING THE HELP YOU NEED AND RECOMMENDATIONS FOR DEALING WITH THESE CHALLENGES

Cultural Barriers

Individual attitudes and responses to mental illness may be highly affected both positively and negatively by one's family and cultural environment.[23] These environments influence the meaning individuals assign, how they make sense of it, what the causes may be, and how much stigma surrounds mental illness. In addition, they affect whether individuals will seek help, from whom, how supportive their families may be, the pathways they take to obtain mental health services, and how well they respond to different types of treatment.

One's culture can sometimes get in the way of one's ability to seek help for mental health problems. In many ways, this has been the case for African Americans. The way we were raised by our family or within our communities often shapes how we express feelings. We sometimes feel uncomfortable talking about problems outside our family—or even within our family. In some families, talking about your feelings or seeking help is considered unacceptable. Mental illness is something that you just don't discuss! As noted in a focus group with women who had received mental health services, "In my family growing up we didn't breathe the term mental illness, even though many of my aunts were depressed and my momma's cousin had been diagnosed with bipolar as a teenager. Momma said, 'We don't air out our dirty laundry to folks.' We sat back and watched them suffer, no medical help at all, I guess they were hoping that Jesus would fix this too!" For these reasons, African Americans may feel that if they discuss their mental health with a professional, they are being disloyal to their families or showing a sign of personal weakness. However, taking care of your mental health is too important to ignore, even if it embarrasses those close to you.

Reliance on Religion/Spirituality

The prominence of spirituality and religion in the African American community also plays a factor in hiding or ignoring depression.[24] Many people who could benefit from professional mental health care are urged to rely on faith and prayer rather than seek out mental health treatment. In many instances, seeking counseling is considered a lack of faith in God's divine healing powers. African Americans often receive the message that one should endure life's difficulties without appearing weak and that their faith should carry them through. But what happens when one sees their problems as larger than "prayer," or if one may not have a religious affiliation? Does one become lost in the dark? As a result, many African Americans have gone without needed care, and when they have sought care it has been at the crisis stage, which is not the most effective way to engage in mental health care. We don't need to limit ourselves to an either/or scenario. Pastoral (clergy) care can occur alongside mental health treatment.

Cultural Mistrust of Medical Providers

Many African Americans remain wary of the medical establishment, so we are slow to seek out care, and particularly including the processes involving mental health treatment. Issues of distrust in the health care system and mental health stigma frequently lead African Americans to initially seek mental health support from nonmedical sources. Often, African Americans turn to family, church, and community to cope.[25]

The 1972 Tuskegee medical study was one of the most horrific acts of oppression that set the stage for generations of mistrust of the American mental health system. "No scientific experiment inflicted more damage on the collective psyche of African Americans than the Tuskegee Study."[26] The U.S. Public Health Service (PHS) conducted a syphilis study in which African Americans and other racial/ethnic groups were used as guinea pigs, and died due to improper treatment. Trusting the idea of free medical care, with no knowledge of the study—these innocent people became victims. It is no wonder that many Black people in this country have trouble trusting the medical establishment.

Lack of Access to Economic Resources

The fact that African Americans disproportionately lack health insurance and often don't have a regular health care provider causes many African American people to seek primary care from the emergency room, where doctors and other personnel often miss diagnoses of depression.[27] In fact, a 2009 study found that two-thirds of primary care physicians were unable to obtain mental health care for their patients who needed it, largely because their patients lacked insurance coverage or the barriers to using it—such as high deductibles and low caps on the number of visits allowed—were prohibitive.[28] Even when we want to take care of our mental health and emotional selves, we don't always have the means to do it. Because Americans consider mental health a lower priority than medical health, not all employers include mental health benefits in their plans, so even those with health insurance may not have mental health coverage, or its deductible may be high or its cap on covered expenses low.[29] As with any professional service, counseling can be expensive, running between $75 and $150 an hour in many areas where African Americans live, although you may be able to join low-cost group sessions and inquire if some providers offer sessions on a sliding scale.

How Can You Find a Mental Health Provider?

Various mental health professions educate and train persons to provide effective mental health services. Some may specialize in certain areas, such as depression, substance abuse, or family therapy. They may work in different settings, such as hospitals, clinics, social service and community agencies, private practice, or other facilities. These professionals may be psychiatrists, psychologists, social workers, psychiatric nurses, licensed mental health counselors, or even professionals from other disciplines. Each profession brings something different to mental health care. Psychiatrists and most psychiatric nurses who offer mental health services are also able to prescribe medication. Other providers, such as social workers, may align themselves with doctors or refer you to a doctor who can prescribe medication if necessary. Clinical social workers can also provide assessment, mental health therapy and counseling, and a range of other services. Clinical social workers offer assessments, diagnosis, and mental health therapy to individuals, couples, families, and groups. They often work in a private or group practice, although many work as therapists or clinicians in settings such as mental health clinics, hospitals, schools, and community centers. Clinical social workers focus on the biopsychosocial aspects of a problem, meaning that they take a "person-in-environment" approach that involves a thorough consideration and investigation of the biological, psychological, and social factors that can affect a person's functioning and well-being. Clinical psychologists offer many of the same services as clinical social workers. They often provide specialized psychological assessments, diagnosis, and psychotherapy to individuals, couples, families, and groups. However, psychologists are also specially trained to administer psychological tests, such as personality and intelligence tests. Psychologists take a slightly different perspective when treating patients, tending to focus more on behavior and cognition than social workers do.

Mental Health Providers: Tips on Finding One

Mental health providers are professionals who diagnose mental health conditions and provide treatment. Most have either a master's degree or more advanced education and training. Be sure that the mental health provider you choose is licensed to provide mental health services. If you've never seen a mental health provider before, you may not know how to find one who meets your specific needs.

Below are some points to keep in mind as you search for a mental health provider:

- When you go for help with your mental health struggles, it's important to find a place you trust and a provider you feel comfortable working with. You may feel more comfortable with a mental health professional who is a woman or man, or within an individual or support group setting. You may prefer a provider that is close to you in age or has a similar racial or cultural background or religious affiliation.
- The skill of listening is important in identifying a provider. You want to find someone who is a good listener, someone who lets you come up with your own ideas, who'd keep your business to themselves and won't be frightened by your feelings. If you have that person and as a result of talking with them you feel better and make positive changes, that's a great move. If not, you are free to find another provider who meets these needs for you.
- Most mental health providers treat a range of conditions, but one with a specialized focus may be more suited to your needs. For example, if you have an eating disorder, you may need to see a psychologist who specializes in that area. If you're having marital problems, you may want to consult a licensed marriage and family therapist. In general, the more severe your symptoms or complex your diagnosis, the more expertise and training you need to look for in a mental health provider.
- Consider whether you need medications, counseling, or both. Some mental health providers are not licensed to prescribe medications. So your choice may depend, in part, on your concern and the severity of your symptoms. You may need to see more than one mental health provider. For example, you may need to see a psychiatrist to manage your medications and a psychologist or another mental health provider for counseling.
- Consider your health insurance coverage. Your insurance policy may have a list of specific mental health providers that are covered or only cover certain types of mental health providers. Check ahead of time with your

insurance company, Medicare, or Medicaid to find out what types of mental health services are covered and what your benefit limits are.

To find a mental health provider, you have several options:

- Seek a referral or recommendation from your primary care provider.
- Ask your health insurance company for a list of covered providers.
- Ask trusted friends, family, or clergy.
- Check to see whether your company's employee assistance program (EAP) or your student health center offers mental health services.
- Check phone book listings or search the Internet under categories such as therapists, counselors, psychologists, psychiatrists, social workers, or social service organizations.

What should you look for in a mental health provider?

- Don't hesitate to ask lots of questions. Finding the right match is crucial to establishing a good relationship and getting the most out of your treatment.
- Education, training, licensing, and years in practice—licensing requirements vary widely by state
- Areas they specialize in and specific services they offer
- Treatment approaches and philosophy
- Office hours, fees, and length of sessions

HOW TO TALK WITH PROVIDERS ABOUT TREATMENT CHOICES

Consumers are encouraged to ask questions of their providers' treatment perspectives and intervention methods. Do not be afraid to ask questions about your provider's treatment perspective, and do not just assume that what you are hearing is correct. Have a list of questions handy. Your health is the most important of your possessions. It is important to feel that your provider is competent so that you can relax knowing you are in "good hands." Additionally, at the start of treatment, you and the provider should agree upon the changes you want to make in your life, a realistic time frame for achieving them, and how you will know when change is achieved. Then you begin working together toward achieving these changes. After a few visits, you should know if you're working with someone who is committed to and invested in you making the change you want and is most appropriate to help you meet your goals. If you are not feeling comfortable and safe, then no matter how good that provider may be, he or she may not be good for you.

You should bring a notebook with a list of questions that you would like answered. You are also encouraged to share your preferences, values, and beliefs regarding medicines and medical care. A few suggested questions that you may want to ask appear below:

1. What are the recommended treatments to address my depression? What are the risks and benefits associated with the recommended treatment?
2. What are the goals of the treatment being recommended? How long will it take before I feel changes?
3. What should we do if problems get worse or we do not see an improvement?
4. How will the recommended treatment promote my strengths?
5. Is there research showing that the recommended treatment works for African Americans?
6. Have you worked with African Americans seeking treatment for depression before?
7. How can I reach you after hours or in the event of an emergency?
8. Is the recommended treatment covered by my insurance, and what is the cost?
9. Are medications available to me to treat my depression? What are they, and what are the side effects?

WHAT ARE THE TREATMENTS THAT MIGHT HELP ME?

Although depression can be devastating and life altering, it is highly treatable. In fact, more than 80 percent of those diagnosed with depression are effectively treated and return to their normal daily activities and feelings. Mental health care can help you feel better and enjoy life again. However, it is important to note that there isn't one type of mental health care; there are many. "Talk therapy," traditionally known as psychotherapy, is not a unified field. Accordingly, providers, whether a psychiatrist, psychologist, or social worker who provides counseling or therapy, may use a number of different approaches and techniques—namely, cognitive behavioral, interpersonal, and family systems. Each of these approaches has a unique perspective on what causes people to suffer from depression and how best to fix those problems.[30] However, all mental health care approaches and techniques aim to teach individuals about their depression; help individuals understand, express, and control their feelings more effectively; and transform negative thoughts, attitudes, behaviors, and relationships. The best mental care for you will seek approaches and techniques that depend on the type of problem you are facing. It may be one-on-one therapy or counseling. This is when you talk with a doctor, a therapist, or a counselor alone. Family therapy, on the other hand, is where various individuals of your family are a part of your care. Your provider may suggest that you bring in a family member or friend. Another option is to join a group, where you talk with other people like yourself along with a provider. Your doctor may prescribe medicine to help control or reduce your symptoms. These treatments can be used alone or in combination. Additionally, attention to lifestyle, including diet, exercise, and decreased smoking and drug use, can result in better physical and mental health.

Talk Therapy

Individual therapy allows you to meet with your therapist and identify those issues and feelings that interfere with daily life. This is especially useful when you have a history of hurt and disappointment, trauma, physical illness, or loss. How you perceive and process those experiences can alter your relationships with others, affect your long-term health, and cause you to waste a lot of life opportunities.

Taking the time to get an objective understanding of your strengths and flaws can make you so much stronger. Having a neutral, trained professional with no fear of your changing for the better can give you the confidence to try new ways of being. The value of therapy is that people often make *permanent* changes in their thinking and then practice skills that reduce problem behaviors and thoughts with no side effects and no long-term health concerns. There are many benefits to therapy that are emotional, financial, physical, and spiritual.

Group Work with African Americans

It has been suggested that group practice with African Americans provides a less stigmatizing and more empowering context for help-seeking than other forms of mental health treatment.[31] Support groups are used to affirm the nonnurturing, hostile social and psychological realities and to offer the opportunity to assist one another in coping with the consequent psychological distress. Further, African American support groups provide the opportunity for African Americans to explore themselves as a whole personal being. In a group setting, African Americans may have an immediate sense of camaraderie, a sense of belonging, a shared history, and an opportunity for personal growth with support for (1) clarifying their identity as a person, as an African American, while looking at how this affects one's relationships; (2) identifying one's concept and image of oneself; and (3) dealing with roles that one plays and stereotypes that hamper the full expression of self.

Medication Can Be Helpful

Therapy and counseling strategies have been developed for many mental health disorders and can be used without medications for patients with mild or moderate depressive symptoms. However, if a person is experiencing increasing and unrelenting depression to a point where he or she can't identify the source, then the combination of medication with therapy has proven to be most effective.[32] Medications don't permanently cure everyday emotional discomfort, but some may reduce depression in a way that really helps. However, in my work with African American women, they expressed a preference toward the use of talk therapy over medication. In our conversation regarding the use of medication to help ease depressive symptoms, Shelia shared her experience. She stated, "I would try to talk to him about what's wrong and the first thing he would do was pick up the pen and let's go Abilify, oh Zoloft, oh dededadaa. At one point I was on like six medications, all based on the recommendation of my so-called psychologist, and what bothers me is that I go to the appointment to try to talk to him about what's wrong with me and all he can say is, 'Let me see the psychiatrist about writing you a prescription.' That's all they do, they don't even listen to what I have to say deep down inside."[33] The women voiced tremendous frustration that practitioners were not genuinely interested in hearing about their concerns but prescribed medication in lieu of supportive counseling. While we understand that medication is an important foundation of treatment for patients with more severe symptoms, we must be aware of their feelings and experiences about the prescribing of psychotropic medication; sometimes it helps just to ask prior to proceeding.

There are many types of medications that have been developed to do different things to treat depression. You might be prescribed an antidepressant or antianxiety medication. If you are being treated for moderate to severe depression, a doctor or psychiatrist may prescribe an antidepressant medication for you. The side effects of antidepressants can cause problems at first, but then generally improve with time. One way antidepressants work is by altering the balance of certain chemicals in your brain.[34] And as with all medicines, this change can cause side effects. Some, like increased anxiousness or restlessness; nausea or upset stomach; weird dreams, inability to get to sleep, or difficulty staying asleep; and diarrhea, typically go away after two to three weeks. If they don't, it's probably best to switch to another drug. Others, like dry mouth or decreased sexual desire, may last longer.[35] Not everyone has the same side effects, and a particular antidepressant doesn't cause the same side effects in all people. You shouldn't feel abnormal, awkward, or self-conscious if you have any of these side effects. You should, however, talk to your doctor about them—especially if they make you feel worse or the side effects themselves are unbearable. Whatever you do, do not try to manage your medication on your own. Do not suddenly quit taking your medication, because it could cause intense withdrawal symptoms or even a return of your depression. You need to talk to your doctor before making any changes to your medication. With time, you should find the benefits of treatment outweigh any problems from side effects.

In order to get the most out of medication, consumers must make an informed choice about taking medications and understand the potential benefits and risks, as well as costs, associated with medication use. In addition, they must take the medication as prescribed by a mental health care professional. Deciding when medication is a better first step rather than therapy depends on several factors, most primarily the urgency and the intensity of emotional pain or when one is engaging in unusual or harmful behaviors. *ALERT!* If a person is suicidal or has suicidal/homicidal thoughts, they need immediate hospitalization, even if they tell you they are "okay." People can even fool themselves about their capacity for self-harm or harm of others. Encouraging them to go to the emergency room for an evaluation or supportive care is the best advice one can give.

EVIDENCE-BASED TREATMENT APPROACHES FOR DEPRESSION

What Are Evidence-Based Practices?

Evidence-based treatment has seen a growth in the development of new therapies over the last twenty-five years. When the term *evidence-based practice* is used to describe a treatment or service, it means that the treatment or service has been studied, usually in an academic or community setting, and has been shown to be effective in repeated studies of the same practice conducted by several researchers across the country.[36] The studies typically use uniform training and a treatment manual to guide providers in the treatment. They also provide supervision and oversight to help ensure that providers follow treatment procedures as outlined. While evidence-based therapies are not perfect treatment approaches by any means, they may represent the best that the field of mental health currently has to offer consumers.

Consumers generally appreciate the direct approach to treatment taken by many evidenced-based treatment approaches, but some will benefit from a more traditional, free-flowing, or less-structured mode of therapy.[37] It is just fine to follow a more structured, evidenced-based treatment approach with a more traditional supportive therapy, or to participate in both evidenced-based treatment and supportive forms of care at the same time if these options prove helpful or useful to you.

Cognitive behavioral therapy (CBT) and interpersonal therapy are two evidence-based treatment psychotherapies that have documented success in treating people with depression. CBT is a type of therapy that helps consumers understand and modify thoughts and feelings that influence behaviors.[38] CBT is based on the idea that negative actions or feelings, such as those associated with depression, are the result of current distorted beliefs or thoughts, not unconscious forces from the past. Interpersonal therapy focuses on the personal and/or social relationships of the depressed person. The idea of interpersonal therapy is that depression can be treated by improving communication patterns as well as understanding each other's actions, feelings, and behaviors and how they are able to relate.[39] As with medication, not all people with depression will be helped by evidence-based therapies. Keeping this in mind, we conclude our discussion of evidence-based therapy approaches to treating depression with brief introductions to culturally responsive perspectives that can also be helpful when working with African Americans.[40]

Self-Help Strategies

Given that African Americans are less likely to have access to "comforts"—such as mental health services—there are several alternative self-help and community interventions that can make dealing with depression easier. We must accept the fact that there are some forces beyond our control—from political realities to painful budget cuts—creating stressors that undermine our mental and emotional health. These facts of life we cannot change. But we can control our responses to these situations, including committing ourselves to protect our emotional well-being and to restore our psyche when it succumbs to an assault. The key to overcoming depression is to start with a few small goals and slowly build from there. Draw upon whatever resources you have. You may not have much energy, but you probably have enough to take a short walk around the block or pick up the phone to call a loved one.

Come up with a wellness toolbox that includes things that you can do for a quick mood boost. Include any strategies, activities, or skills that have helped in the past. The more "tools" for coping with depression, the better. Try to implement a few of these ideas each day, even if you're feeling well:

- Keep stress in check. Not only does stress prolong and worsen depression, but it can also trigger it. Figure out all the things in your life that stress you out. Once you've identified your stressors, you can make a plan to avoid or minimize them in your life.
- Eat a healthy diet, and exercise daily. A balanced diet that includes fruits and vegetables can boost your mood and make a difference in your energy levels. Take a long walk, ride a bike, or work in your garden—every minute counts!

- Visit friends or family. Often, when you're depressed, it feels more comfortable to sink into your shell, but being around people you enjoy and love will make you feel less depressed.
- Make a phone call to a family member or good friend. Share what you're going through with the people you love and trust, and ask for the help and support you need. The people you talk to don't have to be able to fix your problem; you just need them to listen.
- Avoid alcohol and drugs. If you're using alcohol and drugs to cope, you could actually make your symptoms worse, both while you're using them and in the long run. Be careful with the mix of alcohol or drugs and medications; they can be deadly.
- Sleep well. Depression typically involves sleep problems. Whether you're sleeping too little or too much, your mood suffers. Get on a better sleep schedule, aiming for at least eight hours a night.
- Practice relaxation techniques. You'll be surprised by how just relaxing reduces stress. A daily relaxation practice can help relieve symptoms of depression and boost feelings of pleasure. Try taking a hot bath, or practicing yoga, meditation, or deep-breathing exercises.
- Do the things you enjoy. When you're feeling down, it can make it really hard to get motivated to do the things you love. Try to make yourself do one thing you usually enjoy each day. Read a good book, watch a funny movie/TV show, or listen to relaxing music.

When self-care becomes a regular part of our life, we create an environment where the mind/body/spirit connection can really kick in. Make sure that you are eating balanced, regular meals; getting out to exercise; varying your routine to include fun activities; and sleeping eight hours daily. Below you will find suggestions for you to keep in mind for your Wellness Toolbox:

- Keep stress in check.
- Eat a healthy diet, and exercise daily.
- Call or e-mail a family member or good friend.
- Avoid alcohol and drugs.
- Expose yourself to sunshine.
- Practice relaxation techniques.
- Visit friends or family.
- Sleep well.
- Do the things you enjoy.

CULTURALLY SPECIFIC TREATMENT
PERSPECTIVES AND APPROACHES

The field of mental health has recently paid more attention to the needs of African Americans through culturally responsive practice approaches. These methods equip providers with cultural knowledge about racial and ethnic groups to increase cultural literacy and to improve the level of understanding that mental health care providers bring to their work with clients from different cultures.[41] Although this attention is a step in the right direction, it overlooks the importance of developing and using practice interventions that reflect the lived experiences of African Americans. Culturally responsive counseling practice requires an ethic of understanding in an effort to build bridges between persons whose cultures and backgrounds do not necessarily mirror mainstream America. Hence, culturally responsive counseling refers to the inclusion of diverse perspectives in the counseling process in a manner that validates and affirms persons from marginalized groups and recognizes the contextual dimensions of race, culture, class, gender, religion, sexual orientation, and geography.[42]

There are two models that many African American researchers and providers have identified as methods central to improving mental health services for understanding depression among African Americans in mental health care: the Africentric and Black feminist perspectives.

AFRICENTRIC PERSPECTIVE

Africentricity is a dynamic perspective, derived from "diverse lived experiences,"[43] that not only views human interactions based on principles of equality but also considers the connections that exist between the major social divisions of race and class. The concept of Africentricity was introduced by scholars in the 1970s as a response to the neglect of African people in America.[44] Over several decades, researchers and providers have argued for the development of alternative social science models reflective of the cultural background and cultural reality of people of African descent.[45] The objective of the concept was to reconstruct the African American identity through the development of theories and practice frameworks that reflect and affirm the values and worldviews of African Americans in the social sciences literature.

Africentricity is both theory and practice that is rooted in a cultural orientation toward spirituality, interpersonal relationships, communalism, and expressive communication.[46]

Africentricity provides a framework for understanding the importance of the social context and informs the use of culturally competent interventions.

Africentric intervention methods may be culturally appropriate when working with African Americans because they give guidance and purpose to the understanding of problem behaviors and suggest appropriate solutions.[47] For example, for an African American male who abuses substances, it is the aim of an Africentric intervention to engage him in a process of raising consciousness about and affirming his cultural identity, and to revisit traditional problem-solving and coping strategies from a cultural perspective.[48] This positive identification with African American culture fosters resilience and creates opportunities for social and psychological change to occur.

An understanding of the Africentric perspective serves as a blueprint for navigating the complex and culturally unique life circumstances that often lead African Americans to seek mental health care. The integrated perspective suggests that working with consumers from an Africentric point of view creates a space where African American consumers feel supported and valued. It fosters a sense of positive racial and/or cultural identity that creates a social context in which clients can benefit from mental health care and apply new coping strategies.[49]

The Africentric perspective is most valuable if it is infused throughout the mental health care process. It facilitates engagement because it enables the clinician to communicate an understanding of African American values that is likely to engage clients. It informs a more thorough assessment process because it provides a framework for understanding the importance of social context in determining outcomes. It is also critical for intervention because it informs the process of using strategies that are designed to foster a sense of racial pride.

THE BLACK FEMINIST PERSPECTIVE

It used to be said that African American women didn't realize they had depression because they lived their lives never expecting to be happy. Hopefully, that's changed with new generations of sisters welcoming all the joy and opportunity that they can find. Even with these great expectations, they are often confronted by a host of challenges, which need to be met with a plan. African American feminist scholars and practitioners adopted an urgent mandate to address all forms of inequality and oppression through a Black feminist perspective.[50] The Black feminist perspective consists of processes and methods that offer more complex understandings of gender and its intersections of difference and incorporate a fundamental understanding of African American women's historical, sociocultural, familial, and developmental heterogeneity. This perspective recognizes different ways of seeing African American women's reality from a positive standpoint and helps to forge a greater understanding of their strengths, resilience, and struggles.

African American feminisms in mental health treatment are not a set of therapeutic techniques, but rather a lens in which to view the world, a value of responsiveness, and a political and aesthetic epicenter that informs practice.[51] However, there is consensus among many African American feminist therapists about some of the structural elements of the therapeutic process. Structural elements include, but are not limited to, a negotiation of fees, accessibility of space, minimization of power differentials, acknowledgment and valuing of African American women's experience, recognition of the impact of the multiple oppressions on the consumer's experience, and sensitivity in the naming and diagnosing of problems/issues.[52] African American feminists have also restructured the practice of therapy through the deep integration of consciousness raising, exploration of their multiplicative and compounding life stressors and circumstances, race-gender role analysis, backing of the prioritizing of self-care over that of others, insistence on not minimizing one's pain, strategizing against competing life demands, and the exploration of how African American women's concepts of citizenship affect their political engagement.[53]

For Providers: Culturally Congruent and Responsive Mental Health Care

The history of African Americans in the United States is one of survival, resilience, and collective solidarity despite encountering blatant and implicit forms of discrimination. As Americans continue to challenge the ideologies that support oppressive mental health frameworks, race remains one of the most salient social indicators in our society.[54] For African Americans, the centrality of race impacts daily life and can be both a source of contention and strength. Many African Americans live with environmental discriminatory disadvantages that place them at high risk for behavioral and emotional challenges. African Americans' participation in culturally congruent programs leads to more interaction and expression of cultural norms, which may improve treatment outcomes.[55] Mental health interventions that are culturally congruent may be more compatible with African Americans' cultural experiences and create a supportive social context that promotes holistic wellness.[56]

Culture, which can be understood to be a combination of common heritage beliefs, values, and rituals, is an important aspect of racial and ethnic communities. African Americans are a resilient people who have withstood enslavement and discrimination to lead productive lives and build vibrant communities. Throughout U.S. history, the African American community has faced inequities in accessing education, employment, and health care. However, strong social, religious, and family connections have helped many African Americans overcome adversity and maintain optimal mental health.

African Americans and European Americans share many values an
as do individuals from many other cultures. However, there are ⌐
factors that should be accounted for in working with many African American
clients. It must also be noted that African Americans are a diverse group and
that individuals vary by social class, religion, region, and education. Culturally congruent strategies ensure that mental health treatment is effectively
addressing the treatment of psychosocial needs of African Americans and
their families.

The culturally congruent and responsive practitioner's task is twofold: to
help clients know and appreciate the impact of culture in their lives and to
help them act in empowering ways by challenging unhelpful cultural assumptions and external societal biases. Practitioners must be ready to welcome the multiplicity of difference that African Americans bring to the treatment process, and at all times invite them to draw on their experiences.

As practitioners engage with African Americans, they might consider the
following strategies for recovery:

- Discrimination, racism, and sexism are societal realities for many African
  Americans. Acknowledge these societal oppressions, and allow consu-
  mers to identify their own experiences.
- Family is often broadly defined as extended networks of family members
  and friends; include family and ancestors as sources of pride and support.
- Spirituality and religion are highly important and integral for most African
  Americans; practitioners should allow consumers to draw on these contexts as a coping mechanism.
- Proactively build trust and engage in empathy in intentional ways. For
  example, be "real" and discuss any racial, gender, class, and/or sexuality
  differences that may exist.

SUMMARY

In this chapter, we have provided relevant information based upon the literature and clinical experience on how to restore and preserve our mental health.
We discussed essential elements to consider as you support someone else in
his or her journey to mental wellness and healing; specifically, identifying
when we need support, understanding treatment access, understanding options for African Americans, identifying potential barriers, and learning how
to choose a provider. It is our hope that you can now with confidence answer
the question, "Are you ready to be well?"[57]

In affirmation, and with the needed skills and tools, we must answer,
"Yes, I'm ready to be well." For instance, your cousin (or maybe niece,
nephew, or brother), who gathered with you over this past holiday season,

displayed a mood of despair, hopelessness, and described himself as feeling "tired and not able to get to class or work." The good thing is that he has just received confirmation from you that there is sun beyond the clouds and that he does not have to suffer alone. You are now aware of many signs and symptoms of depression and are confident in your ability to pull him aside, let him know you care, and assist him in reaching out for the support he needs. The very next time you see him at a family gathering, you see his face full of delight and joy, and you are told, "Your encouragement was felt and heard. I talked to my college advisor, and she referred me to a counselor, one who looked like me, understood me and my struggles with depression. After a few months of weekly counseling and participation in a group led by a 'brotha' that consisted of 'brotha's' I was able to rise above my dark clouds. I just wasn't alone. Thank you, cuz. Thanks for pulling me up, instead of dragging me along."

As a community of African Americans and allies, we must first acknowledge that persons with depression can't just "snap out of it," and getting help for depression is a sign of strength. We need to engage in a sustained and massive effort to eliminate the stigma of seeking mental health services. People need to know that depression is real, depression is treatable, and help is available.

Chapter Three

Dealing with Mental Illness

Community Interventions and Innovative Programs for African Americans

Pamela P. Martin

Linking depressed persons to available mental health services and resources within their own community serves as a mechanism for helping people navigate the fragmented mental health system of care. Traditionally, case managers help with the service and treatment navigation. Widely accepted duties of case managers include eligibility assessment, treatment planning, direct linkages with agencies, recommending available supports to assure needs are being met, monitoring progress, and advocating for improved service provision. However, for some African American families, using the services of a case manager is not possible or is improbable given that the concerned family member wishes to seek assistance for a relative privately. Most often, case managers are not involved in the depression treatment process. When the services of a case manager are not a viable option, a concerned family member must focus on maximizing the depressed person's ability to use available resources to improve functioning. The concerned family member might do the following:

1. Think about how to broker continuity of care (keeping the same doctors in one mental health practice facility or one mental health professional);
2. Maintain accurate medical and medication records;
3. Figure out transportation needs to appointments;
4. Develop a relationship with a pharmacist and pharmacy to monitor medications and dosages;

5. Seek supports for himself or herself because taking care of an unwell person requires energy and patience; and
6. Remain flexible to the ever-changing insurance coverage rules, availability of community programming, and the time it takes to experience improvement.

One of the many considerations that must accompany helping a person seek treatment in the community is understanding how community interventions function and learning what the potential options are.

One critical topic for African Americans seeking depression treatment is to understand the difference between "state hospital" treatment (inpatient care) in the community and receiving treatment using community-based organization interventions (outpatient care). State psychiatric hospitals represented the mental health system for a long time, but what is familiar about the facility is that it is for inpatient care. Most people are familiar with "insane asylums" from over one hundred years ago where psychiatric hospitals served as a refuge for a mix of conditions including mental illness, developmental disabilities, and being homeless. As time progressed, state psychiatric hospitals clarified their role as serving persons with severe and persistent mental illness. While experiencing depression can be considered severe and persistent, due to the high demand of those needing hospitalization, persons with depression are often treated in the community rather than on an inpatient basis. State psychiatric hospitals across the country serve many different types of persons and vary significantly in the services provided. Persons seeking treatment range in age from children to the elderly. Few state psychiatric hospitals provide care shorter than thirty days (acute care). The more typical length of stay serves persons between thirty to ninety days, and for terms longer than ninety days, the average stay is 120 days.[1] Although state hospitals do tend to admit community members actively experiencing the severest distress (e.g., a suicide attempt), persons diagnosed with clinical depression that can be managed on an outpatient basis are unlikely to be hospitalized. What type of community treatment can African Americans expect from their communities?

From the perspective of one of the authors, community interventions need to be understood in consideration of the whole person. The bioecological theory offers an explanation of how mental health   practitioners, mental health advocates, family members, clergy, policy makers, and community leaders, among others, access community resources for people suffering from depression. Specifically, bioecological theory explains the help-seeking behaviors of depressed individuals. These help-seeking behaviors provide evidence that could explain not only the depressed individual's decision making when it comes to reaching out for help but also how various social systems interact with the individual's help-seeking behaviors. As everyday people concerned about their depressed loved ones (as well as mental health professionals/practitioners) use bioecological theory to understand the dynamics of treatment provision in consideration of the person-in-environment, they then can use bioecological theory to explain interactions between developmental growth and those systems.

As professional practitioners seek out ways to assist people dealing with depression, many mental health advocates will use bioecological theory in order to distinguish dynamic interactions between social systems and an individual's developmental growth. In particular, when bioecological theory is used to treat African Americans dealing with depression, the theory helps mental health advocates identify which systems (e.g., educational, financial, judicial, medical, political, etc.) are either helping or hindering access to mental health services among African Americans dealing with depressive symptoms.

The bioecological theory best suited for assessing effective treatment options for African Americans dealing with depression includes five interconnected processes: microsystem, mesosystem, exosystem, macrosystem, and chronosystem. Knowledge about how these five processes constitute a culturally competent, bioecological approach for treating African Americans dealing with depression should offer a solid foundation for the mental health services process. The theory allows the service consumer to critique his or her own knowledge about how members of institutions serving the African American community's mental health establish a pathway for asking questions that will continuously prepare her or him about mental health services. Specifically, African American consumers of community interventions will be able to sort out what resources are necessary to promote positive, psychological well-being most directly affected by persons experiencing depression. Figure 3.1 depicts the bioecological model to show you how each part is integrated.

This chapter provides stories about African Americans dealing with depression to demonstrate how community interventions function and aid in the healing process. Vignettes are used throughout this chapter in an effort to protect the identities of African Americans serving as exemplars dealing with depression while at the same time illustrating the real challenges faced today. Emphasizing challenges in dealing with depression as a part of race-based identities as African Americans, the chapter also reviews the importance of community-based programs that promote positive, psychological well-being. The presented composites allow readers to explore other people's encounters with depression as well as learn how churches, schools, and other service institutions support African Americans who are dealing with depression. The text following each vignette offers a critique of each person's challenges with depression that focuses on their common experiences based on race theory

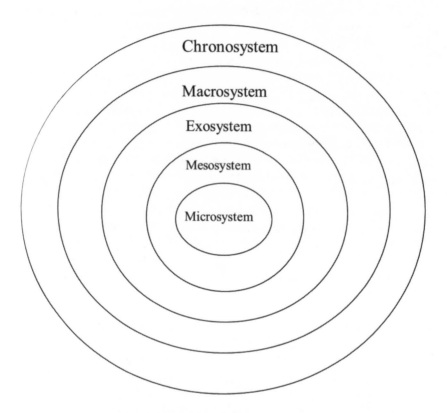

Figure 3.1. Bioecological Model and Depression.

and provides another way for readers to evaluate what they believe mental health providers and researchers may need to consider.

Readers will also gain a better understanding of how structural factors such as race, gender, and poverty may adversely influence the overall psychological well-being of African Americans already dealing with depression. Lastly, readers will find that this section also provides pastors, ministers/clergy, teachers, school counselors, principals, researchers, mental health professionals, and community members with examples that assist each stakeholder with defining, creating, and sponsoring culturally relevant mental health programs to promote positive psychological well-being within diverse African American communities.

Application Exercise 1: This exercise can be completed either individually or as a group. The questions below will allow the reader to reflect upon and respond to African Americans dealing with depression. Referring to figure 3.1 might be helpful in answering the questions.

1. Considering what you have read in previous chapters, list a few reasons why some African Americans dealing with depression do not seek mental health services.
2. In your own words, how would you describe bioecological theory?
3. How does bioecological theory relate to African Americans dealing with depression?
4. What do you want to learn about depression and community interventions?

IDENTIFYING AND ACCESSING COMMUNITY-BASED INTERVENTIONS AND PROGRAMS

Community-based organizations, families, faith communities, and schools can help identify resources providing services to individuals dealing with depression. Access to effective resources such as interventions and prevention programs takes collaboration from each key stakeholder. The initial step to gain access to interventions and programs is identifying available resources in a local community. For example, there are several national crisis and information call centers that assist individuals with finding mental health resources in a local area, and these call centers target different groups who might be dealing with depression such as adolescents, college students, graduate degree students, postpartum mothers, and veterans. The Internet is also a useful tool to aid in finding mental health resources, such as the Center for Parent Information and Resources, Mentalhealth.gov, and the National Alliance on Mental Illness (NAMI). Each of these resources can assist with helping to locate inpatient or outpatient facilities in a local community. Please refer to the appendix to locate contact information for these organizations.

Community-based interventions targeting depression vary in types of programs offered and treatment outcomes. Depending on the severity of depressive symptoms, individuals seeking to identify mental health services have different options available. Some examples of these programs include mobile crisis centers, crisis and assessment centers, family programs, adolescent treatment programs, and faith-based programs. A brief description of these programs is below.

Some communities offer mobile crisis services as well as crisis and assessment centers. Mobile crisis centers provide a twenty-four-hour and seven-day-a-week assessment and triage service. These centers allow helping professionals to provide services in the community by meeting a person potentially dealing with depression in a safe environment in his or her community, to conduct assessments, to evaluate appropriate services that may be needed, and to provide some crisis stabilization services. A *crisis event* refers to an individual's response to an occurrence that is understood to be threatening, hazardous, or extremely upsetting and is not resolved using available coping skills.[2,3] Crisis and assessment centers employ licensed clinicians who meet and assess treatment needs. Once the assessment is completed, a consultation is conducted to find an appropriate treatment setting before the consumer leaves the center. In most cases, these centers also provide crisis stabilization, if necessary.

Adolescent treatment programs assist youth ion dealing with depression. Examples of services include academic support, basic skill development, individual and group counseling, and family therapy. In these adolescent intervention programs, youth participate in a variety of treatment sessions depending on the individual program and scheduled activities. Activities include, but are not limited to, role playing, cognitive-restructuring techniques, homework exercises, and short quizzes to develop individual coping strategies. Examples of adolescent treatment programs are Adolescent Coping with Depression Course, Coping with Stress Course (CWS), and Prevention of Depression (POD). The Kaiser Permanente Center for Health Research provides free, online access to youth depression treatment and intervention programs, so please refer to the links in the appendix.

Family services programs attempt to aid families by trying to improve the family unit. Many of these services provide parenting programs that focus on topics such as developmental stages of children and adolescents, expectations and goal setting, effective discipline, and family members' roles. When searching for evidence-based family services programs, NAMI recommends practical things such as taking notes and asking questions to identify culturally competent programs that align with the family's own values.[4] Examples of some of the questions NAMI suggests parents ask the provider include:

1. Why are you recommending this treatment, and what are the alternative treatments, if any?
2. How does the recommended treatment promote my child's strengths, capabilities, and interests?
3. Is there research showing that the recommended treatment works for families like ours?
4. What are the risks and benefits associated with the recommended treatment?[5]

Please refer to the link in the appendix regarding NAMI's *A Family Guide— Choosing the Right Treatment: What Families Need to Know about Evidence-Based Practices*.

Faith-based interventions allow individuals to use their faith as a coping resource to deal with depression. Bible study, worship services, life skills training, and counseling in treatment sessions are used in these programs. In the African American community, faith communities historically have provided valuable support to congregants and the broader society. Some community-based organizations have begun to partner with African American faith communities to assist in training providers to become more familiar with the diversity within African American communities. Partnerships between faith-based organizations and community providers also use existing services already offered by many African American faith communities, such as transportation, meeting space, and respite care. Recently, the Hogg Foundation has begun to fund and investigate mental health initiatives within African American faith communities.

For individuals who want to become mental health advocates, the Community Tool Box (http://ctb.ku.edu/en) provides a free, online resource to promote overall community health and to create positive societal change. The Community Tool Box, created at the University of Kansas, offers forty-six chapters and sixteen related tool kits of community-skills building that help individuals become advocates who promote local, state, and societal change.[6] Some examples of the tool kits in the Community Tool Box consist of creating and maintaining partnerships, assessing community needs and resources, developing strategic and action plans, and sustaining the work or initiative.

Microsystem and the Immediate Environment

The microsystem contains the influences of significant people who compose an individual's most immediate environment (e.g., the family) and the ways in which those people interact with the genetic makeup of the individual dealing with depression. In essence, the microsystem reveals the human forces at work within the immediate, surrounding environment of individuals dealing with depression. For African Americans who are depressed, the microsystem might include a number of people who are active in his or her life that have shaped and impacted the navigation of the immediate environment; more precisely, the microsystem could reveal the people who actually are willing to offer help and serve as ones from whom help is accepted. It is assistance from these people that may be more likely to cultivate relationships with mental health professionals who serve their communities. In contrast, some African Americans dealing with depression will go to great lengths to conceal their need to ask for help, an avoidance that may adversely impact psychological well-being.

For African American adults dealing with depression, the microsystem includes social interactions found in families, health care organizations, mental health services, religious congregations, and civic as well as social groups. For some depressed African American adults, their microsystem also shapes daily functioning compared to just their encounters with other people. For African American children or youth dealing with depression as well as living with an adult exhibiting depressive symptoms such as their parents, siblings, extended family members, and/or their peers, any or all of those persons are potential influences in the microsystem, and, as such, their influences may impact the social, cognitive, and psychoeducational development.

Microsystem and the Family

Similar to most families, many African American families hold particular beliefs about which behaviors lead to optimal physical and mental health not only for themselves but also for the members of their family such as children, youth, and elders. These beliefs usually attempt to integrate the family's traditions, customs, and value systems in order to communicate messages to family members about overall well-being and good health. Researchers assert that many African Americans are collectivist (i.e., communal), wherein they underscore the significance of interdependence, which can be demonstrated in relationships created and maintained by extended family and fictive kin networks.[7] Extended family members include aunts, uncles, cousins, and grandparents, whereas fictive kin includes precious relationships with non-blood-related friends, affiliations with fraternity or sorority members, and dependence on mentors or role models like coaches and teachers. Moreover, many African American families that employ a collectivist approach might have their blood relatives who are not a part of their nuclear family share in significant responsibilites such as financially contributing to the rearing of children, providing consistent or occasional child care, and taking care of elderly family members. These extended family members along with the family's network of fictive kin participate in numerous rites of passage such as baptisms, birthday celebrations, graduations, weddings, funerals, and extracurricular activities like children's soccer games or nonprofessional sporting events. Moreover, one national study reported that African American families also may use their fictive kin relationships to assist in other, individual circumstances beyond rites of passage. Consequently, social scientists have endorsed the possiblity of family and friends becoming allies in order to encourage African Americans dealing with depression to seek mental health services. In a study by Heller and colleagues, researchers reported that family members and friends accurately predicted depression among a sample of elderly women regardless of race.[8] Heller and colleagues also examined the extent to which mental health programs meant to assist with and address issues of depression intentionally promote the involvement of extended family members and fictive kin network.[9] The vignette below provides an example of an individual family dealing with depression at the microsystem level.

Why Is My Mommy So Sad? Postpartum Depression

Mrs. Shante Jenkins, thirty-two, a married mother of two boys who lived in an affluent community in Atlanta, Georgia, agreed with her husband, a successful engineering professor at a prominent Atlanta university, that after the birth of their second child, Shante would leave her job in finance and become a stay-at-home mom. Shante's mother, although supportive of her daughter's determination to provide her children with a full-time mother, constantly worried about Shante's decision to give up a lucrative career and her own professional ambitions. Neither Shante nor her husband ever regretted their decision, but they were somewhat surprised when they realized they were about to go through their third pregnancy. Unlike Shante's previous pregnancies, she could not muster any feelings of attachment for their child and only girl, whom they named Elise. After giving birth to their little girl, Shante cried frequently, experienced bouts of insomnia, had a hard time concentrating, and also started to have disturbing thoughts. Shante shared her feelings with her doctor, expressing both guilt and shame for not being as emotionally connected to Elise and also for not being a good mother to their daughter, as she had been for their sons.

Research studies have found that African American women have higher levels of depressive symptomatology than White women.[10,11] Scholars who study postpartum depression explain that these findings may not accurately describe African American women's experience with postpartum depression.[12] Specifically, studies have recruited mothers from low socioeconomic backgrounds who disproportionately tend to be women of color.[13] As a result, researchers need to begin to conduct studies that account for diversity within African American communities, including varied economic statuses. For instance, social support networks, either positive or negative, may have direct relationships on how African American mothers may seek resources when facing postpartum depression. A study by Taylor and colleagues found that demanding relations with kin networks were related to depressive symptoms and were negatively linked to self-esteem and optimism.[14]

Although Shante's story shows signs of postpartum depression, available research indicates that not too much is known about this type of depression among affluent African American women. This story also looks into family dynamics and roles, especially regarding work and self-worth. It also underscores that Shante sought medical help rather than see a mental health provider for her postpartum depression.

Application Exercise 2: This exercise can be completed either individually or as a group. The questions below will allow the reader to reflect upon and respond to situations involving African Americans dealing with depression. Referring to figure 3.1 might be helpful in answering the questions.

1. In your own words, how would you define microsystem?
2. Which details would you list to specifically identify microsystem(s) in Shante's story?
3. What is an extended family? What are fictive kin networks?
4. Are you a part of fictive network(s)? Please provide details to explain your response, especially how you provide assistance for those persons and how other people provide support for you.
5. Based on what you read in previous chapters, what causes depression?
6. How would you explain why research studies about postpartum depression have focused much more on women from lower socioeconomic status instead of middle-class or affluent African American women?
7. Which resources or services in your community provide help for women experiencing postpartum depression?

Charlene's Life Transition

Charlene Carter, a sixty-seven-year-old college professor and married for thirty-five years, was excited about her upcoming retirement plans to travel with her husband. Since she had been working for close to fifty years, Mrs. Carter immediately began to volunteer with several organizations, and initially found them fulfilling. She started to think daily about her life, focusing on her accomplishments as a mother of two successful children, a grandmother of five, and her former successful career. Eight months after retiring, Mrs. Carter became overwhelmed with despair and experienced uncontrollable crying. She avoided calls from her sister-friends, a group of women Mrs. Carter met with once a month for dinner for more than fifteen years. Ben, her husband, became worried about her mental health. Ben made an appointment with Mrs. Carter's primary care doctor, and the doctor referred her to a psychologist. Mrs. Carter was hesitant to see the psychologist, but over time, she began to open up about her feelings. Mrs. Carter currently sees her psychologist, Ada Ponds, once a week. Mrs. Carter commented to her husband, "Dr. Ponds understands every aspect of my life—personally, socially, culturally, and economically."

Depression among senior citizens reflects a major public health concern about the elderly. One study found that African American elders were less likely to be treated for depression than non-Hispanic White senior citizens.

Therefore, help-seeking behaviors among older African Americans dealing with depression play an important role in understanding social support needs within this population.

Application Exercise 3: This exercise can be completed either individually or as a group. The questions below will allow the reader to reflect upon and respond to situations involving African Americans dealing with depression. Referring to figure 3.1 might be helpful in answering the questions.

1. In your opinion, why is retirement a difficult transition period for some people?
2. Which community-based interventions do you believe might be helpful for Mrs. Carter?
3. How might Mr. Ben Carter help his wife transition from career to retirement?
4. Why is Mrs. Carter's sister-friend network important to her overall mental health?
5. How would you describe the ways extended family members and fictive kin networks can partner with mental health programs in order to assist and address various issues associated with African Americans dealing with depression?

Microsystem and Faith-Based Organizations

Service institutions created by and often for African Americans tend to have a broad focus that operates multiple functions. With regard to faith-based organizations such as churches, these African American (i.e., Black) institutions often address a combination of issues that may include social, material, educational, spiritual, and emotional needs. With a nod to the Black family, researchers have pointed to African American churches as the second most significant socialization institution within African American communities after the Black family. Throughout the history of African Americans in this country, Black churches have been the cultural center or foundation of African American communities. Even today, Black churches remain the second most significant social institution in African American communities because after the family, Black churches were the first social institution owned and operated by African Americans.[15]

According to nearly a century of research on African American communities, religion has provided a framework for navigating life experiences, transmitting moral values, and socializing group members via a unifying doctrine. Many if not most of these research studies examine religious behaviors among African Americans, reports of high levels of religious involvement, and recurring religious activities. In sum, African Americans tend to be more religiously active than other groups as they persistently draw upon religious teachings and intentionally cultivate religious behaviors, such as regular church attendance, all in their efforts to create coping strategies. The following story depicts how some Black churches respond to mental illness with silence as opposed to with direct interventions for African Americans dealing with depression.

David's Death: When Suicide Happens

David Henderson, a twenty-nine-year-old African American Christian, failed to attend his weekly Wednesday night choir rehearsal. Aware of David's weekly participation, several church members immediately called but were unable to reach him. Then, the following morning, David did not report to work, so his girlfriend and his mother went over to his apartment. They found David's body in his bedroom. He was dead as a result of a self-inflicted gunshot wound. Devastated, confused, and traumatized by David's suicide, his family, friends, and coworkers struggled to understand David's decision to commit suicide. Janice Brown, his girlfriend, admitted that she was aware of his manic depression. She never pressed the issue regarding medical or professional help since David always reassured her that he would be fine, or she would notice eventually his efforts to just shake it off. David's girlfriend saw his intentional actions to deal with depression on his own as evidence that no further interventions or assistance were needed.

Throughout U.S. history, our entire society—especially public opinions that have been created or influenced by mass media—has encountered stereotypes of African American males that portray this demographic as devoid of those admirable qualities associated with respectful, hard working, problem-solving providers and protectors, qualities which are personified by their Caucasian counterparts. Due to these societal stereotypes, African American males often experience racial profiling, institutional racism, societal inequalities, systemic discrimination, and police brutality in nearly all the regions of U.S. society throughout their entire lives. Furthermore, these documented, lifelong experiences of negative confrontations within U.S. society may cause some African American males to score below average on a number of social indicators regarding mental health, such as exhibiting depressive symptoms and having fewer opportunities to develop healthy coping strategies.[16, 17] Thus, for some African American males, who live in places where violence is a daily reality, there are too few opportunities to develop healthy mental habits like positive self-esteem. To cope with these persistent societal stressors, some African American males may engage in self-destructive behaviors, with an outcome (or intention) being suicide.[18] Researchers confirm that young African American men's access to firearms has led to an increased number of suicides. Several studies reveal that suicide among young

Black men has increased dramatically over the last thirty years and that the majority of these suicides resulted from self-inflicted gun wounds.[19,20] Some of the factors leading to suicide attempts include depression or other mental disorders, drug or alcohol abuse, and domestic violence or a family history of suicide.[21,22] Although initial research studies about suicide among African Americans focused on unemployment and poverty, the singular argument that economic disadvantage is responsible for suicide does not sufficiently explain the increased rate of suicide among African American males. The fallacy is apparent because African Americans who reside in middle-class, predominately White neighborhoods also have seen an increase in the rate of suicide.[23,24]

With an increased rate of suicide among African American males, many Black churches not only have to help their congregation members face the realities of suicide, but equally as important, these Black churches also have begun to address other issues among African Americans dealing with depression. It is not surprising, therefore, that some African Americans have come to rely upon their churches to provide various interventions and programs that promote healthy psychological functioning. Those congregation members now expect some level of assistance with comprehending and reducing the stigma African Americans dealing with depression might experience.

Historically, as the second most reliable social institution owned and operated by African Americans outside of their families, Black churches persistently have provided institutional agency within African American communities.[25,26] Within an incessant context of racism that has plagued African American life in this country, Black churches have provided cultural centers and foundations to neutralize (or negate) the effects of racial discrimination upon/within African American communities. In fact, Black churches have been successful in assisting African American communities with resisting the dominant and destructive forces from largely White mainstream U.S. society. Such success is due to the fact that many African American denominations intentionally were developed independently of White authority or affirmation in contrast to other institutions serving the African American community, such as schools, hospitals, financial institutions, or insurance companies. For these reasons, Black churches are equipped to transform and to educate their congregations about strategic options that promote positive psychological well-being among African Americans dealing with depression.

David's story highlights the increased use of guns to commit suicide and how significant people in his life failed to understand his depression. This story integrates previous sections to help individuals understand the signs as well as the symptoms of depression. David's suicide also should encourage readers to discuss the overlap between mental health issues and religious faith. Refer to the questions below to delve deeper into David's story.

Application Exercise 4: This exercise can be completed either individually or as a group. The questions below will allow the reader to reflect upon and respond to situations involving African Americans dealing with depression. Referring to figure 3.1 might be helpful in answering the questions.

1. How can someone learn to identify the warning signs of suicidal behaviors?
2. How can faith communities promote and develop mental health initiatives to combat depression?
3. What services or community resources would improve the quality of mental health services in your community?

A Pastor's Theology: Does Theology Matter?

In a tight-knit community located in the midwestern state of Michigan, the pastor of a Black megachurch begins his announcements by having his congregation pray for family, friends, and other affected people after the unexpected and tragic loss of a fellow member, Brother David McBribe. After sharing the news of David's suicide, Pastor Smith then asks his wife to stand up and address the congregation by sharing her own testimony about her own battles with depression. He proclaims, "The Lord brought us through this dark episode as we covered our marriage with prayer and fasting. If you seek Him first and place your hope not in this natural world but claim your victory yet to come, I know anyone can overcome a little sadness."

Moore questions how theological teachings at some Black churches seem to promote the stigmatization of depression.[27] According to several theologians and scholars, laypeople and those individuals who may not have exhaustive knowledge about theology often need a much easier way to make sense of the ways theology can influence behaviors among African American believers.[28,29,30] One way of explaining theology's influences in the lives of African American Christians entails discussing the relationships between theology and behaviors in terms of a continuum of influence. At one end of the continuum of influence, the theology of otherworldliness teaches people the universality of the Gospel message and that believers should concentrate their efforts and energies on interpreting the sacred text of the Bible in order to understand how to live a life that focuses on their salvation, their preparations for the afterlife, and their cultivation of moral values. The theology of otherworldliness promotes a frame of reference about reality that discourages active participation in social change efforts because otherworldliness theology does not promote believers getting deeply involved in the affairs of the material world since they should be really concerned about the "other" world, which is their eternal life.

At the other end of this theological continuum, this-worldly theology encourages active participation in efforts to challenge any or all conditions that make life in the United States difficult or dangerous for African Americans. This-worldly theology, for example, empowered the preachers, freedom song singers, and protestors as well as demonstrators and boycotters during the civil rights movement. In other words, this-worldly theology emphasizes African American experiences in U.S. society as an opportunity for interpreting biblical text as both symbol and prophetic affirmations that influence Black people in the United States to seek and fight for mental, physical, and spiritual liberation from oppression. Consequently, some African American theologians explain that this type of Black theology not only engages Christians in social change efforts, but, like otherworldly theology, it also socializes African American congregations about their salvation, their sanctification, and their morality, just with a greater emphasis on the practical and immediate implications of all those spiritual dimensions in the right here and right now.

The "Does Theology Matter?" vignette focuses on the diverse religious messages communicated at Black churches. Although African Americans engage in different faith practices such as Buddhism, Islam, voodoo, and others, the majority of African Americans participate in Christian faith communities.

Application Exercise 5: This exercise can be completed either individually or as a group. The questions below will allow the reader to reflect upon and respond to African Americans experiencing depression. Referring to figure 3.1 might be helpful in answering the questions.

1. With a historical perspective, how would you describe the role of religion in the lives of African Americans?
2. Moore argues that theological teachings at some Black churches promote stigmatization of depression. Do you agree or disagree? Give an example to support your answer.
3. Should faith communities provide mental health outreach services? Explain your answer.
4. How can faith communities partner with other service institutions to promote positive psychological well-being? Name the potential partnering service institutions. Why do you think these institutions would be effective partners with faith communities?

Microsystem: Schools—Mixed Messages
Impairing Psychological Well-Being

Marcus Jefferson is a forty-year-old noncustodial father who has been actively engaged in his son's, Jarrod's, life. Jarrod, a thirteen-year-old middle school student, is underperforming in school, and his teachers characterize his behaviors as disruptive, angry, and responsible for putting Jarrod at risk for failing yet another grade. Although his father monitors Jarrod's activities closely so that his son will not begin to participate in counterproductive behaviors such as joining a gang or selling illegal drugs, the father still feels that his own incarceration for ten years has created a nearly impossible impasse in his attempts at parenting Jarrod. Due to the tensions at school and home, Jarrod, his dad, and stepmother have begun counseling. They are uncomfortable with the psychologist because he only asked presumptuous questions, such as how long have your mother and father been living together. Mr. Marcus Jeffersonwas offended by the question because he recognized the race-based assumption about African American intimate partner relationships. Consequently, the continued presumptions of questions revealed the psychologist was not familiar with African American culture. Despite Mr. Jefferson's best efforts to protect his son from negative neighborhood and peer pressures, Jarrod's behaviors constantly take his son farther and farther away from the productive path Mr. Jefferson is trying to provide for his son.

The incarceration of African American parents disrupts their relationships with their children, undermines the support systems they rely on for helping them with their children, and then creates subsequent child-rearing burdens on extended families, churches, schools, and juvenile courts, as well as health and human service agencies.[31] Researchers suggest that children's exposures to potentially traumatic events, such as the familial disruptions caused by incarceration, are associated with higher levels of clinical problems and long-term physical and mental health outcomes such as depression.[32,33] In short, the incarceration of parents or adults responsible for child rearing threatens the well-being of impacted children, including their mental well-being. Couple these findings with their residence in high-poverty urban areas, and children in these environments experience not only mental health difficulties but also academic underachievement, at elevated rates.[34,35]

Throughout U.S. history, parents and other adults responsible for imparting values to younger generations have stressed the relationships between academic achievement and financial success when it comes to securing an overall high quality of life. However, for many African Americans, special education has compromised their academic achievements, isolating them in classroom settings especially created for learners with difficulties. Over the last several decades, numerous research studies have documented disproportionate numbers of African American males as the target population for special education programs.[36,37,38]

Research also reveals that African American male students who believe there is a discrepancy between what they experience in their own homes or neighborhoods and how they are treated within school environments risk feeling anger, hopelessness, and inadequacy as a result of those differences.[39] Furthermore, African American males who do not see their cultural values and norms being reflected in their academic learning environments may feel as if they do not fit in with their school's culture and are much more likely to have negative relationships with teachers, to drop out of school altogether, and to engage in delinquent juvenile behaviors.[40] African American male students do notice discrepancies between their personal interactions outside of their classrooms and the expectations or perceptions of them in classroom settings.[41,42,43] As a result of the negative impacts of those discrepancies on African American male students, education scholars underscore the pressing need to link effective pedagogical strategies to both historical and contemporary social contexts that can position African American male students to benefit from classroom curricula.[44,45] Specifically, these education scholars believe that culturally relevant curricula will highlight the contributions of African Americans in U.S. society, allowing all students, particularly African American males, to learn in context (i.e., referencing current societal systems such as political, educational, and financial to demonstrate curricular competencies that link back to classroom instruction).[46] Summarily, empirical studies predict dire consequences for such youth, explicitly highlighting risks common to African American males who miss out on academic achievement such as a lifetime of extreme, unrelenting poverty, as well as many types of negative mental health outcomes.[47,48,49,50]

In addition, these education scholars explain that, since classroom teachers come from diverse backgrounds, people concerned about the educational outcomes of all students must understand that classroom teachers' beliefs, expectations, and attitudes about achieving and underachieving students might include stereotypes about African American male students. In effect, teachers' characteristics (i.e., gender, socioeconomic status, and race), their personalities and belief systems, as well as the student-teacher relationship influence academic outcomes. Classroom teachers can also create learning environments that potentially place African American male students in academic settings that either recognize the students' capacities to achieve or facilitate academic underachievement. Consequently, proponents of culturally competent curricula assert that the pedagogy in urban school districts should place the culture of the community at the center of educational processes.

Furthermore, a body of research has documented that classroom teachers hold lower expectations of African American male students' academic achievement regardless of the teachers' racial classifications.[51,52] Although the research shows that African American teachers hold slightly more positive views about African American students, public school teachers' overall perceptions of African American male students remain extremely low.[53,54] Wood and colleagues found that teachers' biases and lower expectations regarding African American male students may persist as students age over time.[55] Some research underscores that teachers' negative expectations contribute to low academic performances among African American male students. With these dire predictions from research findings, culturally responsive teacher training has captured the interests of psychologists, educators, and other community stakeholders who have questioned teachers' pedagogical practices.

Jarrod's story shares the plight of the recent trend among some African American families with a former or current parent(s) being incarcerated. This vignette also discusses challenges many African Americans, especially males, face trying to obtain a quality education. The narrative hints at the point that many African American males are being prepared either for low-paying employment opportunities or for penal institutions by the educational system. These outcomes might lead to hopelessness and despair not only for male students but also for his family, as in the case of Jarrod's father. Finally, this vignette emphasizes the role of teachers in promoting positive psychoeducational development of students.

Application Exercise 6: This exercise can be completed either individually or as a group. The questions below will allow the reader to reflect upon and respond to African Americans experiencing depression. Referring to figure 3.1 might be helpful in answering the questions.

1. What are the microsystems in this scenario?
2. Should schools play a role in providing and supporting the mental health needs of students? Explain your answer.
3. What advice would you give Mr. Jefferson regarding Jarrod's behaviors?
4. How are neighborhood factors such as violence contributing to Jarrod's behaviors?
5. If you could develop a community program targeting adolescents like Jarrod, how would you bring together parents, teachers, police officers, and other important community stakeholders?
6. What are programs in your area helping adolescents similar to Jarrod?

Microsystem: Community Health Centers

A finding from the Centers for Disease Control and Prevention (CDC) found that African Americans were less likely to seek help from mental health professionals compared to the general population.[56] A potential explanation for this finding is access to comprehensive health care among African Americans. A report from the Kaiser Commission on Medicaid and the Uninsured indicated that 21 percent of African Americans were uninsured and 33 percent used a government/other public insurance program.[57] Furthermore, Medicaid provides slightly over half of the health care services for African American children.

Boutin-Foster and colleagues explain that community health centers (CHCs), serving as a critical safety net, offer care for a substantial percentage of vulnerable, medically underserved individuals.[58] Thus, CHCs represent a significant immediate environment for African Americans dealing with depression seeking mental health services. CHCs provide comprehensive medical services for uninsured and low-income children, the elderly, individuals, and families residing in rural and urban areas. The services at CHCs include inpatient, outpatient, home-based, school, psychosocial rehabilitation services, and community-based programs. CHCs along with local health departments and public hospitals serve many economically disadvantaged African Americans for physical and psychological health issues.

One Mom's Journey: Seeking Help for Her Child

LaTonya Jordan is a single mother of two adolescents—Tony, an eighteen-year-old, and Nia, a sixteen-year-old. LaTonya works two part-time jobs to provide for her household. Ms. Jordan's household income is slightly below the poverty line. She has worked hard to provide for her children to do well academically, such as computers and exposing her children to a variety of activities. Both of her children are honor students, testing into a prestigious science and mathematics high school in the suburbs, and she is extremely proud of their hard work. Tony and Nia are extremely close, and although competitive with each other, they help one another overcome difficulties by listening to grievances and offering advice. Ms. Harris, a high school counselor, noticed Nia has begun to have a difficult time concentrating in her classes and has been irritable in class, snapping at several different teachers. Recently, Nia's grades have steadily declined. Ms. Harris met with Nia, and at first the meeting was going well. Suddenly, Nia emotionally shut down and shouted profane words at Ms. Harris. Shocked by the encounter, Ms. Harris scheduled a meeting with Ms. Jordan to suggest she seek counseling for Nia outside of the school. Nia's mother took off work and scheduled an appointment at the Jefferson Community Health Center. At Nia's request, she met with the only African American psychologist at the center. After several sessions, the psychologist concluded that Nia's anxiety and depression stemmed from uncertainty about her future. Tony will be the first person to attend college in his family, and he will soon leave his job at a fast-food restaurant. Since the age of sixteen, the income Tony earned partially contributed to the household income. In preparation for Tony's transition to college and the subsequent loss of household income, Nia resented having to give up extracurricular activities to work and to take over Tony's financial commitment to the family.

Application Exercise 7: This exercise can be completed either individually or as a group. The questions below will allow the reader to reflect upon and respond to African Americans experiencing depression. Referring to figure 3.1 might be helpful in answering the questions.

1. What are the microsystems in this vignette?
2. What are community health centers? Why are community health centers a significant organization in the microsystem?
3. Describe the socioeconomic experience in which the Jordans live. In your opinion, do you think Nia is suffering from depression?
4. What does underinsured mean? How are uninsured and access to health care related?
5. In this vignette, is it appropriate for a parent to expect his or her adolescent to assist in contributing to the household income? Please explain your answer.
6. To what extent can community health centers capitalize on developing outreach efforts and creating programs to include environments such as peers, extended networks, faith communities, educators, medical professionals, and more to promote positive psychological well-being among African Americans dealing with depression?

Mesosystem: African Americans Dealing with Depression

Mesosystems refer to the interconnectedness of the different microsystems working together to support or hinder the quality-of-life experiences among African Americans dealing with depression.[59,60] Depending on the age of the individual dealing with depression, interactions among the different parts of a person's microsystem will represent distinct, immediate environments. For instance, recent findings from the CDC found that women and people residing below the poverty line were more likely to report depression. These findings indicate the multiple demands of women such as parenting, working, and taking care of an elderly relative may contribute to depression. In this study, people dealing with depression are not seeking medical attention. These findings do not address the intersection of race, poverty, and gender in the report. Therefore, African American women dealing with depression whose income falls below the poverty level will need to be identified and provided mental health assistance to help them recover from this particular health concern. Moreover, important community institutions such as family, faith communities, medical facilities, and social services need to continue or begin to create programs that identify and provide services accessible to African American women dealing with depression.

If these findings were unpacked using Application Exercise 7, the different microsystems plus significant individuals either positively, negatively, or a combination of both influencing the person dealing with depression will need to be identified. In this vignette, some of the different microsystems shaping Nia's behavior include single-family background, work, and school. Examples of significant individuals who either positively, negatively, or a combination of both influencing Nia would represent the mother, brother, guidance counselor, psychologist, and Nia's employer. For instance, the description of the sibling relationship represents a positive interaction shaping Nia's development. An example of a negative interaction is the parent-child relationship, which is fostering Nia's resentment. Next, the relationship among different parts of the microsystems and how they work together to impact the daily experiences of dealing with depression will need to be explained. These relationships would comprise mother-daughter, siblings, school and student, medical professional and client, as well as work and employee. Taken together, these interactions help Nia to navigate and cope with the daily stressors in her life. A study conducted at the University of Illinois found sibling relationships have an influence on socioemotional development. In most cases, siblings model behaviors to each other on how to negotiate their immediate environments such as schools, faith communities, and the neighborhood. Research also documented parent(s) as the primary socialization agent that plays a significant role in instilling values in their children.

Application Exercise 8: This exercise can be completed either individually or as a group. The questions below will allow the reader to reflect upon and respond to African Americans experiencing depression. Referring to figure 3.1 might be helpful in answering the questions.

1. Select one example from Application Exercises 1, 2, or 3. What are the different microsystems influencing the person dealing with depression using the vignette selected?
2. Who are significant individuals in the main character's life? Do these important individuals influence him or her positively, negatively, or a combination of both?
3. How do the different microsystems work together to shape the daily experiences of the main character?
4. If you had to identify a community-based intervention, how would you begin to select resources for the main character?
5. What is the Community Tool Box? How can individuals along with community-based organizations begin to create change in schools or medical settings?

Exosystem: African Americans Dealing with Depression

Exosystems represent different social environments that African Americans dealing with depression may not participate in but are impacted by those environments. These environments influence the depressed individual's development by interacting with a structure or structures in his or her microsystem.[61-62] To illustrate, using Application Exercise 7, Ms. Jordan's workplace schedule of having two jobs serves as an example. Tony and Nia are not directly involved in planning their mother's work schedule. Another example in the workplace is the wages Ms. Jordan receives from her two jobs. Both of these situations impact her adolescents' development, and in particular for Nia, she has begun to show symptoms of depression. Neither Tony nor Nia has any involvement with their mother's work and does not assist in the decision making of their mother's work schedule.

Application Exercise 9: This exercise can be completed either individually or as a group. The questions below will allow the reader to reflect upon and respond to African Americans experiencing depression. Referring to figure 3.1 might be helpful in answering the questions.

1. Select one example from Application Exercises 4 or 5. What are the exosystems influencing the main character in the vignette?
2. If you had to identify a community-based intervention, how would you begin to select resources for the main character?

Macrosystem: African Americans Dealing with Depression

Macrosystems, the fourth level of the bioecological theory, consist of the cultural patterns and values that influence the other ecological systems. The macrosystem encompasses the cultural environment in which the person lives and all other systems that affect the person. Examples could include the economy, cultural values, and political systems. The macrosystem can have either a positive or a negative effect on a person's social-emotional development.

Using cultural values as an example, U.S. society and mass media have a long history of stereotyping African Americans. As stated earlier in this section, African American males are perceived as violent, disrespectful, unintelligent, and athletically superior, whereas African American women have been characterized as Mammy, Aunt Jemima, Gold Digger, Welfare Queen, Sapphire, and Diva. Such caricatures depart from the qualities that U.S. society recognizes to maximize the achievements of Caucasians and other ethnic minorities, and this discrepancy often leads to discrimination and racism, which may result in depression. Moreover, historical confrontations with institutional racism, societal inequalities, and discrimination represent a macrosystem for African Americans. Thus, African Americans experience those difficulties in almost all societal institutions across their developmental life spans.

Potential pervasive attitudes among some medical and mental health professions represent an example of the macrosystem. Cultural values in the form of stereotypes might interfere with access and care for African Americans dealing with depression. Research investigating bias among physicians found that some physicians perceived African Americans as less intelligent, less educated, and more likely to have problems with alcohol and drugs.[63] Moreover, another study found that nurses shared similar biases as physicians. The consequences for African Americans concerning quality of care adversely affect treatment and diagnosis. Thus, U.S. cultural values, unless challenged, continue to reinforce stereotypes and behaviors that negatively impact African Americans' daily experiences.

Application Exercise 10: This exercise can be completed either individually or as a group. Questions below will allow the reader to reflect upon and respond to African Americans experiencing depression. Referring to figure 3.1 might be helpful in answering the questions.

1. Referring to Application Exercise 6, what are some examples of cultural values in the macrosystem?
2. How would you explain the ways persistent societal stressors such as race-based stereotypes can lead to depression for some African Americans?
3. Using previous sections, what are some misconceptions about African Americans living with depression? Explain to what extent you think these misconceptions are related to macrosystem cultural values about mental health.
4. How can individuals along with community-based organizations begin to have conversations about racial bias in medical settings such as hospitals, emergency rooms, therapy sessions, and more?

Chronosystem: African Americans Dealing with Depression

The chronosystem represents particular periods of time and developmental shifts that influence a person over his or her life span.[64,65] Additionally, throughout the life span, significant cultural events influence each generational peer group. The bioecological model captures change over time throughout the chronosystem life span. The historical context of the Vietnam War and disco era represents maturing adults, as well as post–World War II, which birthed the baby boomer generation. The founding hip-hop generation such as Sugar Hill Gang, Run-DMC, MC Lyte, and LL Cool J is an example of the chronosystem, and subsequently the neo hip-hop generation includes T.I., Little Wayne, Nicki Minaj, and Drake.

The hip-hop founding generation grew up watching the aftermath of Vietnam through the mental struggles of war veterans. We now know that significant numbers of Vietnam veterans suffered from undiagnosed/untreated depression and related mental impairments such post-traumatic stress disorder (PTSD). As some of those Vietnam veterans became parents, their children, the founding generation of hip-hop, came of age within a U.S. society saturated by street drugs and prescription medication. Whether it was the abuse of Prozac or Valium or hard-core drugs like cocaine, heroin, and LSD, any one of these could lead to self-medication in order to conceal depression among this generation of African Americans. The stigma associated with depression has persistently discouraged African Americans dealing with depression to openly seek treatment during those time periods. The neo hip-hop generation would fall victim to questionable collaborations between public school systems, multinational pharmaceutical corporations, and prescribing health care providers. Each of these collaborators received monetary benefits from the overmedication/unnecessary medication of children and adolescents. Never before in U.S. history have our children been a targeted consumer for drugs. As a result of this historic development, U.S. society has succumbed to a pharmaceutical option to treat any or possibly all ailments including depression.

Application Exercise 11: This exercise can be completed either individually or as a group. The questions below will allow the reader to reflect upon and respond to African Americans experiencing depression. Referring to figure 3.1 might be helpful in answering the questions.

1. After reading this chapter, what is your definition of the ecological model and each system?
2. Select any Application Exercise. What are the depressive symptoms of the main character?
3. If you were concerned about the main character's psychological well-being, what steps would you take to get him or her access to treatment?
4. In general, how would you explain the ways persistent societal stressors such as race-based stereotypes lead to depression for some African Americans?
5. Using the Community Tool Box, how can individuals along with community-based organizations begin to create change in schools, medical settings, and other settings?

Collaborations: Institutional Partnerships

The emphasis in this chapter has so far been upon presenting vignettes of African Americans dealing with depression. Next, this section provides specific examples of community interventions and innovative programs to promote positive psychological well-being within diverse African American communities. Although these examples are brief and hardly exhaustive of the many types of effective programs available in African American communities, it is important to call more public attention to the ways different service institutions are attempting to address and enhance overall psychological well-being among African Americans.

National Alliance on Mental Illness

Health promotion programs targeting African American churches have been successful in addressing several chronic medical conditions such as cancer, diabetes, obesity, and hypertension. Recently, mental health organizations, researchers, and foundations have intentionally called for African American churches to add mental health education or outreach to their health ministry programming. For example, the National Alliance on Mental Health (NAMI) is the nation's largest grassroots mental health organization dedicated to building better lives for the millions of Americans affected by negative mental health.[66] NAMI advocates for access to services, treatment, support, and research and is steadfast in its commitment to raise awareness and build a community of hope for all of those in need. NAMI promotes interventions and programming for faith communities in particular. In so doing, NAMI intends to improve faith communities' capacities to educate their congregants about mental health. For example, FaithNet, one of NAMI's programs, is a network partnership that includes NAMI, NAMI state organizations, and NAMI affiliate leaders and focuses on mental health recovery, resources for clergy, reading lists, and programs as well as presentations.

Mental Health Ministries

Mental Health Ministries, founded in 2001 by Rev. Susan Gregg-Schroeder, a United Methodist minister who has personally experienced living with depression, is an interfaith outreach resource targeting faith communities to reduce the shame and stigma associated with depression. This advocacy organization provides faith communities with a downloadable study guide titled "Mental Illness and Families of Faith Study Guide: The Challenge and the Vision, How Congregations Can Respond," which shares information with clergy, congregants, family members, and individuals wanting to comprehend strategies to respond with compassion and care for people living with depression.[67] It also provides faith communities with a five-step, nonlinear program to create caring congregations about depression. The focus of this program is to meet the needs of congregations so they can develop a more an effective mental health ministry. The five steps are education, covenant or commitment, welcome, support, and advocacy. Other resources available through the website include free, downloadable worship resources; video clips; support groups; books; and information on suicide.

National Suicide and the Black Church Conference

Similar to Mental Health Ministries, the National Suicide and the Black Church Conference was created after a personal experience with depression. In the case of the National Suicide and the Black Church Conference, a female congregation member committed suicide on her church's property.[68] This incident led Bishop William Young and his wife, Pastor Dianne Young, to found the National Suicide and the Black Church Conference. This conference aims to inform different community stakeholders regarding suicide and suicide prevention among African Americans. Under the leadership of the Youngs, Emotional Fitness Centers were created to serve the community in helping to promote positive psychological well-being. These centers attempt the following: (1) to address emotional issues that lead to mental breakdowns; (2) to ensure those needing emotional healing receive it; (3) to reduce the number of people not receiving the emotional help they need; and (4) to lower stress on families associated with family members not receiving needed care.[69] Presently, there are ten Emotional Fitness Centers in Memphis, Tennessee, and two satellite centers, one in Bolivar, Tennessee, and another in Southaven, Mississippi. The programs offered at these centers include prescreening for emotional distress, mental health referral, prescreening for physical symptoms, anger management, and family violence and youth forums.

ParentCorps

ParentCorps, a research study at New York University, examined young children from disadvantaged communities as they began to enter school. This universal intervention brought together two stakeholders important to the academic success of children: parents and teachers.[70] This family-centered, school-based preventative intervention uses family cultural values and beliefs to help parents comprehend and incorporate a new set of parenting strategies to improve the psychological and educational development of their young children. The teacher component of this intervention assists with informing teachers about strategies that address and underscore the diverse needs of children, especially children bringing different skill sets entering school. The teacher component also engages early childhood teachers in strategies that create enhanced, quality classrooms that support social and emotional skills and early learning of students.[71] This intervention, facilitated by trained school staff and mental health professionals, consisted of a series of thirteen group sessions for parents and children held at the school during early evening hours. Laurie Miller Brotman, PhD, the principal investigator of ParentCorps, commented, "Rich or poor, urban or rural, every parent wants their child to succeed. There are hundreds of studies that show that parenting under stress can lead to negative outcomes for children. Parents who are struggling to make ends meet, parents who experience depression, parents who are raising children on their own—all need extra support in their important role as parent."[72]

In summary, this family-centered, school-based preventative intervention reported that parents used evidence-based parenting strategies, used more effective discipline strategies, and were more engaged with their children during play interactions. Teachers rated children in ParentCorps to be better behaved in the classroom and to show more social and emotional competencies, which can potentially lead to better learning outcomes.[73]

The Fathers and Sons Program

Mental health professionals, community stakeholders, clergy, and others interested in promoting positive relationships between African American fathers and their eight- to twelve-year-old sons who are not living in the same home may use or suggest the Fathers and Sons Program. This program was implemented in an attempt to strengthen bonds between fathers and sons. In far too many African American families, fathers do not reside with their children. Research studies show that the lack of a positive father-son relationship may contribute to violent behavior among adolescents, early sexual encounters, substance abuse, and poor academic achievement.[74] Each of the aforementioned behaviors may adversely influence health and psychological well-being. Thus, developed as an innovative, culturally relevant, theoretically based intervention, this program aims to prevent substance use, violent behavior, and early sexual initiation among sons, as well as to enhance healthy behaviors for both fathers and their sons. Additionally, this program involves the local community at multiple levels, including in the design, implementation, and evaluation of the program through participation on the project's steering committee and in dissemination efforts through local businesses. Caldwell and colleagues, researchers from the University of Michigan who created this program, incorporated into the program three themes: effective communication, cultural awareness, and skill building. The curriculum included the following topics over the course of fifteen sessions: Diversity among Families, Culture and History, Health Enhancement Strategies, General Communication, Family Functioning, Parenting Behaviors and Relationships, Using Computers to Communicate, Communication about Risky Behaviors, Culture and Health, and the Closing Graduation Ceremony. Between sessions, the fathers and sons complete homework assignments. The program has forty-five contact hours plus a booster session for graduates. According to Dr. Cleopatra Caldwell, principal investigator of this program,

> The impact of males in a community reaches beyond the roles of father and provider. They also serve as role models, mentors, and forces for social control. When a dad takes a kid to the ball game, he often takes other kids along. Having men in the neighborhood has a balancing, normalizing effect on how kids see the world.[75]

ROSE Program

Caron Zlotnick and colleagues created the Reach Out, Stand Strong: Essentials for New Moms (ROSE) Program.[76,77] This program included four ninety-minute weekly group sessions and a fifty-minute individual booster session two weeks after delivery of the intervention program. ROSE employs interpersonal therapy and is focused on improving social support, familial communication, and factors associated with perinatal depression and major depression among women across ethnic groups.[78] The results of this intervention reveal better postpartum adjustment at three months postpartum than the women who did not receive the intervention.[79]

SUMMARY

The above composites, community interventions, and innovative programs should provide interested stakeholders with information to begin a discussion or plan programs to inform individuals about mental health challenges. More specifically, the intention of this chapter is to highlight structural conditions and to share effective interventions with clergy, policy makers, parents, community activists, and teachers, so that collectively we can provide more effective and culturally relevant mental health services to African Americans. Targeted community interventions and innovative programs can promote positive psychological well-being for African Americans dealing with depression. In discussing these types of interventions and programs, this chapter intends to transform readers into becoming engaged stakeholders who seek to understand how some African Americans deal with depression. Acting as an informed participant in the healing process can only enhance awareness of how depression affects individuals, their loved ones, and their communities. In closing, new knowledge can only empower and place their experiential insight into a problem-solving context.

Chapter Four

Paying for Treatment

U.S. Health and Mental Health Policy

Julia F. Hastings

A just health care system improves the well-being of *all* Americans equally. The new expansions in insurance coverage policy for the American public health care system represent steps in the right direction to support calls for health equity as well as eliminating disparities in access, health outcomes, treatment, and follow-up care. However, gaps remain in unfair ways that divide health care and mental health treatment for African Americans.

Case Study 1

Michelle is a twenty-eight-year-old married mother of two. She has a very demanding, high-stress job as a certified nurse assistant in a mideastern city. Her caseload increased from six patients to twenty. While she enjoys taking her time with each of her patients, she needs to work a little faster to make sure everyone is cared for. Last month, Michelle learned that her health insurance policy for her family had increased the premiums from $400 to $750 per month. Her husband works part time making deliveries. Michelle has always been very good with her patients and graduated with top honors in college. She has very high standards for herself and can be very self-critical when she fails to meet her goals. Lately, she has struggled with significant feelings of worthlessness and shame due to her inability to perform her job as well as she has in the past. For the past few weeks, Michelle has felt unusually fatigued and found it increasingly difficult to concentrate at work. Her coworkers have noticed that she is often irritable and withdrawn, which is quite different from her typically upbeat and friendly disposition. She has called in sick eight times in the last three weeks, which is completely unlike her. On those days she stays in bed all day, watching TV or sleeping. On weekends, she does not shower and yells at her daughters for leaving the living room messy. Her daughters are ten and fourteen years old. Although Michelle has not considered suicide, she has found herself increasingly dissatisfied with her life. She's been having frequent thoughts of wishing she were dead. Her husband thinks she is showing signs of depression. What should he do to begin seeking help for Michelle?

At the end of the day, individuals who seek mental health treatment wish to know how to pay for prescribed treatments such as counseling, medication, and changes in diet and exercise without causing personal bankruptcy. Unfortunately, it is difficult to provide a straightforward answer to "How much will treatment cost?" This difficulty lies in the way the U.S. health care system is set up. In most cases, the costs for care are determined by a person's ability to pay—out of pocket or via insurance coverage. At this time, it is frequently a mix between insurance coverage and services billed directly to the individual to recoup the fees exceeding the insurance cap on cost per service performed. Some treatment facilities offer lower costs for care based on a sliding-scale fee structure that may be determined by household size and income. In any case, whether insured or not, and whether that insurance coverage is adequate, there are many ways to find help in order to pay for treatment.

In the text below, we will briefly discuss the U.S. health care delivery system and components of health insurance (private, military, and public). We will conclude with an explanation of how claims are paid.

U.S. HEALTH CARE DELIVERY SYSTEM STRUCTURE

The U.S. health care delivery system represents multiple attempts to reduce medical costs, increase access to care, and improve the quality of care received. Our health care system is divided by public and private entities that often operate independently and, at times, in collaboration with each other. For example, each individual state sets the rules for private health insurance policies that are not covered by self-insured employer plans. States also fund, manage, and pay part of the public insurance costs (Medicaid) and shape its care delivery within that state. On the other hand, the federal government regulates medication development and medical devices.[1] Unfortunately, very little coordination exists between public and private insurance plans to unify the health care system.

Currently, the majority of Americans (54 percent) receive their coverage from private health insurance, with most privately insured individuals obtaining coverage through an employer.[2] Among those with coverage, high out-of-pocket costs can be a barrier to receiving timely care and medications; one estimate is that medical costs are responsible for over 60 percent of personal bankruptcies.[3] Insured individuals tend to enter the health care system through a primary care provider, although with some kinds of insurance (e.g., preferred provider organization [PPO]), individuals may go directly to a specialist. Uninsured individuals are hindered by a lack of continuity in care, visiting community health centers (which provide primary care for low-income, uninsured, and some populations of color) and hospital emergency rooms. Even after the passage of the latest health policy reforms, one in six Americans are uninsured.[4] Payment mechanisms for each type of health service (e.g., outpatient hospital care, prescription drugs) vary widely due to the complexity of the U.S. health care system.

COMPONENTS OF INSURANCE

Private

Employer-sponsored insurance covers about 149 million nonelderly people, which is commonly referred to as "private health insurance."[5,6] Private health insurance has become a permanent feature of employment benefits provided to employees and their dependents. The benefit involves reimbursing the health care provider for the cost of services rendered.[7] For 2014, it is estimated that average annual premiums are $6,025 for single coverage and $16,834 for family coverage.[8] It is important to note that significant variation in annual premiums exists in the United States as a result of the type of employer benefit coverage, cost sharing, and location in which costs for care may vary. The insurance company associated with the employer estimates the overall risk for the cost for health care services among employee groups and then charges monthly premiums to be paid by an individual or his or her employer.

Military Health System

TRICARE represents the military health care system that provides health care services to over 9.5 million individuals in the uniformed services.[9,10] In May 1997, TRICARE (http://www.tricare.mil) was awarded the contract to administer a health care program for uniformed service members, veterans, and their families.[11] Administratively, TRICARE divides the United States into twelve regions, where each region coordinates the health care needs of all military medical treatment facilities.

Public

Medicaid and Medicare were established with the 1965 amendments to Title XIX of the Social Security Act. Both programs are massively expensive and have been the subject of much political discourse concerning financial cuts. Medicaid is the nation's main public health insurance program for people with low incomes and the single largest source of health coverage in the United States, with coverage for over sixty-six million Americans or about one in every five Americans.[12,13] This public medical insurance program is a means-tested entitlement program that is jointly funded by federal and state funds. Each state designs and administers its own program under broad federal rules. As such, income eligibility levels, services covered, and the method for and amount of reimbursement for services differ from state to state. One basic need most people can recognize as essential to a minimum standard of living is medical care.

Medicare, by contrast, is a universal program designed to help the elderly regardless of income status. The Medicare program covers most hospital and medical costs for persons sixty-five years of age and older as well as persons who are disabled Social Security beneficiaries.[14] The questions that constantly surround both public health care programs are, "What type of health care conditions, and how much service benefit (e.g., prescription drugs), should be provided?" Medicare mimics a private insurance plan and has deductibles and copays.[15] Medicare is structured into four parts. Individuals may be eligible for one or more of the parts:

- Part A—Medicare Part A deals with hospitalization and inpatient services.
- Part B—Medicare Part B deals with outpatient services and routine medical care.
- Part C—Medicare Part C or Medicare Advantage is a way to extend benefits of A, B, and D.
- Part D—Medicare Part D deals with drugs. People with very low income get extra help paying for the prescription costs and deductibles in Part D.

Children's Health Insurance Program (CHIP) or the Title XXI amendment of the Social Security Act in 1997 (and reauthorized in January 2010) represents the most recent addition to the American public health insurance safety net.[16] Its implementation has meant that increased numbers of children in the United States have a regular source of health care, including preventative and mental health services. Under current law, CHIP was funded through fiscal year (FY) 2015 as part of the Patient Protection and Affordable Care Act (ACA). Like Medicaid, CHIP is jointly funded by states and the federal government. CHIP's purpose is to enable states to initiate and expand child health assistance to uninsured, low-income children through (1) a new program that meets special requirements, (2) expanded eligibility for children under the state's Medicaid program, or (3) a combination of both.

The delivery of health care via the public health insurance industry involves a multitude of government agencies involved in financing health care, medical and health services research, and providing regulatory oversight for the various aspects of the health care delivery systems.

FEDERAL MENTAL HEALTH PARITY ACT

Mental health services represent a significant part of medical care. For a number of years, mental health treatment was not considered an important part of wellness care—a separation between mind and body conditions. However, many policy discussions have argued the fact that the costs, coverage, and access to mental health treatment are just as important to healthy living as concerns about medical conditions.

The Mental Health Parity Act of 1996 (P.L. 104-204) legislates that employer group health insurance plans, insurance companies, and managed care organizations offering mental health benefits will not be allowed to set different annual or lifetime dollar limits on mental health benefits from medical and surgical benefits.[17] Mental health treatment is to be considered equal to physical health care treatment. In 2010, the passage of the ACA added individual health insurance coverage to the mental health parity legislation. Treatment limitations (e.g., number of visits or days of coverage) that apply to mental health or substance addictions benefits must be no more restrictive than the predominant financial requirements or treatment limitations that apply to substantially all medical and/or surgical benefits. Medicare, Medicaid, and CHIP are not group health plans or issuers of health insurance. They are public health plans through which individuals obtain health coverage. However, provisions of the Social Security Act that govern CHIP plans, Medicaid benchmark benefit plans, and managed care plans that contract with state Medicaid programs to provide services require compliance with certain requirements of the Mental Health Parity Act.[18]

The Mental Health Parity Act of 1996 does not provide

- a mandate for mental health benefits to be offered in health insurance plans;
- coverage for treatment of substance abuse or chemical dependency;
- rules for service charges, such as copayments, deductibles, out-of-pocket payment limits, and more;
- designations for the number of inpatient hospital days or outpatient visits that must be covered;
- coverage in connection with Medicare or Medicaid;

- restrictions on a health insurance plan's ability to manage care; or
- provisions for businesses with fifty or fewer employees.

The principal beneficiaries of the Mental Health Parity Act will be persons with the most severe, persistent, and disabling brain disorders because they are more likely to exceed annual and lifetime benefits.

HEALTH INSURANCE PAYMENT

Individuals with private or government (public) insurance are limited to accessing medical facilities that accept the particular type of medical insurance they carry. Visits to facilities outside the insurance program's "network" are usually either not covered or require the patient to bear more of the cost than would be accrued by receiving services at facilities inside the insurance program's "network." Low reimbursement rates have generated complaints from providers with government insurance and some patients who have difficulty finding local providers for certain types of medical services.[19,20]

HEALTH CARE REFORM IN 2014

The Patient Protection and Affordable Care Act, more commonly referred to as the Affordable Care Act (ACA), signed into law on March 23, 2010, resulted in many significant changes in the U.S. health care system. ACA makes health care more broadly available to those without access to affordable health insurance. The ACA also makes insurance coverage and payments for mental health conditions equal to any health condition. Federal and state-based insurance "exchanges" are established for individuals without access to employer-based insurance and small employers that choose to purchase coverage. The ACA allows providers that organize into Accountable Care Organizations (ACOs) to share in savings they achieved in the Medicare program. The ACA include numerous features affecting private and public insurance coverage, employers, providers, and consumers. Its main provision is expansion of private and public insurance coverage. Other provisions now possible are:

Private Insurance Coverage

- Substantial subsidies (on a sliding scale) toward the purchase of health insurance for individuals and families with incomes below 400 percent of the federal poverty level.
- An insurance requirement that individuals and families have health insurance coverage. If they do not, they pay a penalty unless the lowest-cost

plan available to them has a premium that exceeds 8 percent of the person's income.

- The establishment of federal and state-based health insurance "exchanges," where competing insurers offer their products to individuals and small businesses. The states have much authority over how they will regulate the insurance market. Health insurers will offer a variety of specified benefit packages that must cover essential health services.
- A requirement that insurers provide a guaranteed issue of a policy to any applicant and to renew that policy. They cannot charge higher premiums based on health status or preexisting conditions. Exceptions are that older enrollees can be charged up to three times as much as younger ones and that smokers can be charged 50 percent more than nonsmokers.
- Insurers are also prohibited from placing annual and lifetime limits on the dollar value of coverage.
- A requirement that health insurers return 80 percent (individual and small group) or 85 percent (large group) of premiums in the form of health benefits.

Public Insurance Coverage: Medicaid

- In states that choose to accept federal subsidies (initially at 100 percent of expenditures, declining to 90 percent), Medicaid coverage will be expanded to individuals and families with incomes at or below 138 percent of the federal poverty level.

Case Study 2

Mrs. Hammer is a fifty-four-year-old widow with two teenagers who worked as a short-order cook until she was fifty-three. She began smoking at sixteen years old. She knew diabetes was a possibility, partly because she was a little overweight, but mostly because it runs in her family. She may have even been told she was diabetic by her primary care physician two years ago, but Mrs. Hammer did not wish to check her blood sugar daily, exercise, or eat balanced meals. Mrs. Hammer went to the doctor regularly until after her husband died when she was fifty and she became eligible for Medicaid. While a lot of people can suffer from diabetes for years without recognizing any signs, Mrs. Hammer began suffering numbness in her hands a year ago so badly that she could no longer cook and became unemployed. Last year she developed chest pain and knew she could not tell her daughters about her aches. Every day for a year, Mrs. Hammer suffered in silence. She felt achy, ate unhealthy food choices (e.g., potato chips, French fries, and fried catfish were favorites), slept for eighteen hours a day, and could not remember to pay her bills from month to month. Mrs. Hammer made multiple trips to the local emergency room, but by a rapid assessment she was diagnosed with depression. Her income was only $8,000 last year, so her family was eligible for Medicaid under ACA. Medicaid paid the emergency room visits and her medications for depression and diabetes when she remembered to take them as prescribed. Mrs. Hammer's costs to Medicaid last year were $800 (six office visits, six group visits for depression services, transportation to her appointments, and medication copays). Unfortunately, should Mrs. Hammer lose her Medicaid benefits because of earning more income—$18,000—the Affordable Care Act will not help her due to the Medicaid expansion rules of her state. What can she do for medical care if she cannot earn a higher income? The answer is she can still qualify for health insurance through her state exchange market. While searching for plans, Mrs. Hammer will be able to compare and enroll in quality health insurance plans and perhaps find an affordable option.

Public Insurance Coverage: Medicare

- A provision that certain preventative services be provided with zero co-payment
- Gradual removal of the "doughnut hole" for prescription drug coverage
- Reduction of government payments to Medicare Advantage plans
- Provision of bonuses to Medicare Advantage plans that achieve high quality scores
- Formation of a board that will make binding recommendations to contain costs (unless overridden by Congress) if fee-for-service Medicare costs grow more quickly than one percentage point above the gross domestic product

DEPRESSION PREVENTION CONSIDERATIONS

Depression rates in the United States are identified as a major public health problem that is growing among African American adolescents, women of child-rearing age, and men (who have been ignored in the past). The prevalence of depression has increased and begins earlier and earlier with each passing generation. The African American population also needs to be aware of the risk factors identified so that attempts to prevent depression symptoms represent a growing research focus. Most mental health resources are currently dedicated to treatment. However, many limits regarding treatment exist, such as (a) services reach very few, especially among needy African Americans; (b) treatment is only effective in about two-thirds of those who follow all treatment directives; and (c) the chances of depression recurrence are 50 percent after one episode, 70 percent after two episodes, and 90 percent after three episodes.[21] It is increasingly necessary to dedicate resources to depression prevention activities. Compared to treatment research, prevention efforts have developed rather slowly.

Prevention activities remain a worthy pursuit because of their potential effects. Delivered in mental health, health, and school settings, these activities deal directly with children, with parents, and with the whole family. Defined by the Institute of Medicine (IOM) report on preventing mental disorders,[22] "prevention activities or interventions occur before the onset of the disorder, and [are] designed to prevent the occurrence of the disorder." As such, resources are used to screen for the likelihood of developing clinically assessed depression.

By contrast, treatment was defined as "interventions occurring after the onset of the disorder to bring a quick end to the clinical episode." Strategies to prevent depression often are designed based on what is known about depression treatment. A considerable amount of scientific study has been and continues to be devoted to learning skills to regulate mood and to reduce symptoms of depression. Four levels of prevention activities are commonly found:

1. Universal preventative interventions
2. Activities that target entire communities regardless of risk; for example, television shows dedicated to identifying symptoms and resources on how to seek assistance
3. Selective preventative interventions
4. Indicated preventative interventions

Experiencing a depressive disorder decreases quality of life, workplace productivity, and fulfillment of social roles. Most research on prevention work occurs among adult populations. More and more research is being devoted to adolescents, adolescents with depressed parents, and school-aged children. The research on reporting the incidence of depression for children younger than age six is not known. It is challenging to assess children for two reasons. First, clinicians are not clear whether symptoms that resemble depression are actually due to depression or are merely developmentally normal difficulties. Second, it is uncertain the degree to which depression is due to developing behaviors of the parent-child relationship or individual experiences. All told, research is still being conducted to understand more about the development of emotion regulation processes during early childhood.

SUMMARY

Historically, prevention has received far less attention than treatment concerns in either mental health or physical health. Current federal policy, research, and practice solutions are scattered across a wide variety of agencies. Research on prevention (and treatment) is organized to address individual disorders and problems, not preventing occurrences. However, there is a silver lining about obtaining treatment. The competition of insurance companies to sway new enrollees just might bring down costs for services and increase access to care for more people. The implementation of the Medicaid expansions within the Affordable Care Act allowed for an additional eight million children and adults to enroll in public health insurance. Fewer people with no insurance represents a good step toward better health.

As for paying for treatment, the price of health care continues to rise. Employers are making changes to insurance policies offered at work that can impact both costs and access to care. It appears as though more responsibility for health care costs will fall to individual workers. African Americans with concerns about their mental health should take advantage of any tools made available by employers to help make informed decisions about mental health benefits and medical care coverage.

In conclusion, the priority in the American health care system should be placed on educating everyone on the best ways to reduce the stigma associated with mental, emotional, and behavioral problems, and on engaging relevant professional and intergovernmental organizations to coordinate care systems. Good health insurance can be expensive. Often, health insurance is out of reach for low- and moderate-income families, particularly if health benefits at work are not offered. In the long run, consideration needs to be given to an effective, broad-based, strong public health approach to improving overall health while taking care of people who cannot afford the rising costs for receiving treatment.

Chapter Five

Concluding Remarks

Finding the Tools to Look Present-Day Chaos in the Face

Julia F. Hastings

Throughout the book, we—the authors—have discussed how to cope with the stressors and symptoms of depression common to modern-day life for African Americans. We all need guidance or a road map, if you will, to sort out all matters around us. More than ever, today's American society faces a variety of issues that strike at the very core of our souls. Thus, this book hopefully serves as a helping resource. We are in the middle of a chaotic time, allowing us to question our existence, relationships, purpose, and life goals while dealing with demoralizing situations. It is easy to feel helpless because online and broadcast news overwhelms us with story after story about tragic events. We are flooded with stories that only make our search for balance farther out of reach. Being unable to attain peace, harmony, and genuine respect as a human being can easily lead to the depths of depression both as a member of a larger community and as an individual.

Currently, some African Americans strain under the load from different pressures that even the most relaxed and reflective person cannot ignore. Depression symptoms loom on any given day. African Americans can experience sleep problems, changes in appetite, display irritability, and exhibit decreased energy. For one individual, these symptoms may be temporary. For another person, these are persistent symptoms that may indicate depression. Although these symptoms are signs of depression, if you talk to any two depressed people about their experiences, you may think they were describing entirely different realities. For example, one might have the ability to maintain his or her usual energy level while the other might feel tired and unable to motivate himself or herself to get up in the morning. Merely living and engaging in everyday life can easily raise questions on how to cope with the burdens. Uncertainty surrounds us, and feeling "depressed," though without a diagnosis, takes on a life of its own. As a result, it is easy to feel lost, ineffective, and sad about not being able to immediately change circumstances for the better.

COMMUNITY COPING DURING TRYING TIMES

Inequality between rich and poor, addictions, shorter tempers, and unplanned persons moving into the home take on larger-than-life roles such that we are swamped with numerous social problems in our lives. The constantly wavering financial highs and lows of America's economics make us struggle with being one paycheck away from the street. Diseases—incurable or not— plague our minds with an unshakable fear that no medication exists for treatment. Rumors of war and terrorism rattle our sense of security as a democracy so much so that it is frightening to explore and travel freely. We can also see problems that affect our loved ones, such as climbing health care rates, natural disasters that force starting lives over, and behaving kindly when actions cause nothing but upset and rage.

Across the country, we learn about events that make us question the very nature of humanity. For example, some African Americans of contemporary times have one time or another thought about why be nice to others who are nasty? When glancing at a person, he insults with a vile term? What is the right way to react? A natural response would be to get angry, irritated, or react in some negative way. However, an appropriate response is many times understood harshly, looked upon as "no home training," and possibly dangerous to the point that life is lost. Reacting in a justified manner for African Americans remains a catch-22. The "right way" appears to be twisted in the details of the story so much so that the event weighs heavily on the mind. Unfortunately, it is part of the American character to worry about who is to blame in times of trouble, and for African Americans, assigning blame takes on an extra emphasis in the mind.

Current events create profound questions for African Americans. The grief and distress of dealing with social status, respect, and the law transforms into the lynchpin of personhood in the changing demographics of U.S. society. It sets us on a different path in terms of dealing with where we fit in the scheme of things. Many African Americans understand events happening across the country through a dual lens: as a citizen and as a member of a culture. This is especially the case when dealing with privileged culture. In the face of tragedy, African Americans have to deal with the outside perception they already face as a racial group. We have extra burdens to work out. When a national tragedy hits home, the media also paints how American society sees us. This same perception can define how we are treated in the workplace, the shopping mall, school, as well as other places we conduct our daily business. Drastic happenings that occur in the larger expanse of the United States can affect our ability for societal access and equity. In 2015, achieving equality, decency, respect, and dignity is more important than ever.

African Americans in society struggle with ethical responses to everyday social problems. Others turn microaggressions into a moment of satire. Still, for some, it is probably easier to ignore what is happening and go on with daily life. The question, "When is it my turn?" rarely gains an answer. The dilemma of simply developing a response to ill treatment turns into its own set of problems for an individual; namely, repressed anger and possible ruminating thoughts about how one would have behaved differently if given a second chance. Sadly, there is plenty to be depressed about when trying to develop a strategy for conquering such barriers.

For African Americans, striving for acknowledgment and kindness turns into a lifelong social practice and easily lends itself to depressive symptoms. An African American's life is laden with indignities on a daily basis. A fear of mistreatment might happen with every situational meeting. Some of those uncomfortable anxieties revolve around being the last served in a restaurant, lingering too long in a place of business, or dealing with the perception that one could be a thief. Even worse, when others mistake an African American as poor and on welfare, such views create more hardships in the public sphere. Even though African Americans are not the only group on government assistance, the stigma of poverty stirs up more trouble for being believed and heard by other people in all levels of society. African Americans branded with the label of being loud, angry, or disrespectful also hinders being taken seriously. The choice of clothes also is scrutinized. The painful lesson learned from mistaken assumptions about personal character is that privilege shields and protects. Those who reside in the realm of institutional and individual privilege do not suffer the same pressure to be accepted by the outside world. Eventually, the need to simply be recognized as a human being changes into a larger movement just to alleviate the distress that lack of personhood brings. The undercurrent for the nationwide protesting and civil disobedience can be attributed to finding an avenue to express unfair practices.

Fighting for societal advancement has reawakened the need to redefine what our community reflects to the rest of the country. The neglectful treatment of police brutality by the legal sectors of the United States especially adds emphasis to the attack on the African American psyche. While seeing the rebirth of fighting for equitable treatment, we have so much to conquer socially as well as individually. Many challenges arrive in our path, questioning our selfhood in the larger landscape of the nation. Every so often, a newsworthy event shakes up the tried-and-true notions, putting African Americans on the stage where our community is being judged by the outer world. On such occasions, we search for answers about where we stand in perceiving what happens around us.

The ability to find clarity is a very important aspect of defining one's self in the midst of society. One can cope with anything when the pieces fall together. It all comes down to receiving the inspiration to fight for change in order to balance one's self and society around them. This is even more important when depression becomes part of the suffering an African American must concurrently experience while stressing out on larger, nation-wide happenings. Attempting to alleviate low feelings transforms into a search for a higher purpose and understanding.

HAVING DEPRESSION IN THE MIDST OF CHANGING TIMES

The single thing that makes depression a unique disease is that it can hit anyone at any time, place, or day. It is rather indiscriminate in its cruelty to an individual. Traumatic events, changes in body chemistry, or overwhelming, profound grief also add tremendous depth to the impact of the disease. Sometimes, an inherited family pattern also plays a part in defining how this terrible illness can strike an individual. The precise cause of depression is hard to pin down. Defining such an illness depends on how it manifests itself in the one who is afflicted. A significant life happening is not the only way to send someone into a long bout of melancholy. To one person, subtle changes can make such suffering just as profoundly horrible. Each person is different. No one can define or uncover which event will do the most damage for an individual. One experience might be positive for a person, while for another the same experience is the worst possible tragedy that could happen. Only you can determine what makes you sad.

Ultimately, we hope that this book is used as a starting point to get better. Knowing what made you upset in the first place helps when trying to embark on a healing course toward wellness. Finding the reasons behind your distress helps in recognizing the triggers leading to drastic and debilitating episodes. Uncovering the truth behind suffering can also help in finding the type of assistance needed when working on recovery. Understanding can also lead to a better insight about the physical changes that depression can bring.

Depressive symptoms are not universal among people. Each person will experience the gruesome effects of this disease on an individual basis. An individual's emotions will dictate how depression will affect life mentally and physically. Melancholic symptoms cannot be easily seen. Hiding in plain sight is a more apt description of depression's behavior. Experiencing the treacheries of feeling sad cannot be compared with a bout of the flu. Instead, changes in attitude or a difference in behavior indicates something is rather wrong. Family members can become complete strangers over subtly mutated actions by a person diagnosed with this awful illness. For example, a person having a vibrant and effervescent sister who loved traveling, living life, and being outdoors suddenly finds his or her sibling transforming into a reclusive shut-in. In the midst of this drastic change, the afflicted builds barriers between herself and others who affect her. She may see that this blockade mirrors a "protective cocoon" from experiencing pain from the outside world. In reality, the lack of concentration and the continued sapping of her vibrancy contribute to her lack of attachment to the outside. Unfortunately, the poor ability to find joy builds a prison instead of the delusion of a haven of safety. During this time, the depressed person also alienates herself from the ones who love her the most as they all try to find the meaning behind this tragic disease.

Sadness is universal for all of us. Everyone experiences feeling down at any given time. Depression, on the other hand, is a different type of experience entirely. Depression cannot be wished or joked away. It is not just the blues, and you cannot just "get over it." Being in recovery takes caring, loving, and understanding individuals willing to help when things end up at their worst. Persons with depressive symptoms often feel alone, rootless, and rather unloved. Without anyone else to listen or aid in the face of such ugliness, this mental illness can inflict its most brutality on an ailing individual—utter loneliness. Because depression has the power of disrupting life, tranquility, and family ties, it possesses enormous staying power for an individual. The enormous depth behind this mental illness causes a battle that is not for the weak willed. Trying to recover from depression takes a lot of courage and heart, which may be hard to find during its worst days. If you have ever experienced depression or been close to someone who has, you know that this disorder cannot be changed at will.

Against tremendous odds, one must find the wherewithal to tap into a resource of empowerment. At first, it takes small steps, for example, sitting up from lying down on the bed or bathing and getting dressed in clothes. As one gains more awareness about his or her bout with depression, the disease can be slowly vanquished one day at a time. In the end, finding resources for help can make having depression manageable. Thus, there is always hope and resilience while coming out of such a dark time.

MINDFULNESS: A TOOL FOR RECONTEXTUALIZING AND REFRAMING

Daily life is filled with anxiety, fear of the unknown, and unexpected events. Naturally, we might experience an influx of emotions when dealing with job loss, drastic medical news, or changes in environment. While it may be easy to give up and let a higher power take over, another way to deal with a highly pressurized situation is to practice mindfulness. To solely work on centering one's mind allows us the opportunity to make a radical shift in personal consciousness. Redirecting attention away from chaos (ruminating thoughts) helps us turn our attention toward being "aware" of the matter at hand and shifting feelings of distress toward calm. Thus, "starving" the anxiety out of a particular situation can lead one to redirect one's energy toward rethinking the situation more positively.

Mindfulness is the practice of being aware without judgment of what is being experienced in the present, both internally and externally. Becoming conscious of how we perceive and respond to life situations means living mindfully. It is not difficult to practice. The key is to change one's attention to a positive focus. Living mindfully shifts our entire way of being. The difficulty is remembering to be mindful. Anyone, including people with depression, is challenged by a "busy" mind. Our thoughts become so absorbed with ideas, memories, perceptions, and other mental fare that it is easy to forget "quieting the inner workings of one's brain" can be helpful and calming. The type of mindfulness that we practice determines the level of balance and calm that can be achieved. The importance of ceasing reoccurring thoughts and focusing toward meditative action requires the ability to resist nervous activity and letting your concerns go momentarily. Practicing this activity while being depressed can especially help in times of agitation.

Experiencing depression tempts the mind to create suffering. The "magnetic pull" of stressful thoughts and feelings renders a person helpless and stuck within the midst of his or her pain. Being stuck represents a mode of stagnation, if you will. The difficulty of doing anything makes the ability to be mindful a challenge for depressed people. In this mind-set, making the shift toward calmness and tranquility can resemble a tug-of-war. However, when one finally achieves the unique moment of peace, it can be recalled whenever a triggering event happens. Practicing mindfulness is important to making progress—a step toward asking for help.

By making mindfulness a habit, learning to give less time to depressive thoughts and actions is improved. Eventually, as it becomes easier to rely on mindfulness as a stopgap measure for easing anxiety, depression ceases to take over and win. Using this method empowers an individual to think more clearly, practice conflict resolution, and take a much-needed break from the weight of heavy thoughts before something drastic and life altering occurs.

LEARNING MINDFULNESS FOR BEGINNERS: THE FIRST STEPS

Below is an easy-to-follow exercise to help develop your mindfulness during difficult situations. Remember, mindfulness takes time to develop, and it will likely be an ongoing process.

- Sit in a quiet room where you won't be disturbed.
- Close your eyes and focus your attention on breathing. It is natural for some to lose attention. When that happens, simply return to focusing on breathing slowly in and out.
- While focusing on breathing, allow your thoughts, feelings, beliefs, and body sensations to enter your awareness as you lesson your focus on things outside your mind.
- Now ask and answer: What are my thoughts, feelings, beliefs, and body sensations right now? Would I describe my current feeling as peaceful?

Using mindfulness as a tool to manage depression symptoms, paying attention to personal experiences rather than being lost in them, means developing a different relationship to individual responses and trigger events. In particular, negative depressive thoughts can be understood for what they really are—just patterns in the mind, arising and passing away, rather than "the truth." Troubling, ruminating thoughts are weakened, and the trapped door to wellness is opened.

WHAT DOES RESILIENT LIVING LOOK LIKE FOR AFRICAN AMERICANS?

When something goes wrong, what happens? Do you press onward in progress? Do you fall apart? Actualizing resilience means using inner strength to meet a challenge or setback. Being without resilience leads to feeling overwhelmed, ruminating thoughts, and sometimes unhealthy behaviors such as abusing alcohol and other illicit drugs. Stating one has resilience does not make problems disappear, but relying on personal inner strength can help in problem solving. Developing skills in being resilient can always be achieved because it is at the cornerstone of the ability to adapt to adversity. It is instituting mindfulness. Tips for improving African American resilience include:

1. Building strong, positive relationships with others. Positive social support will build strength to hold the intention to not judge yourself or

others. As others offer more support, you will find yourself kinder and more supportive of others.

2. Increasingly accept the *facts* of a situation *rather than* your *feelings* about a situation. In other words, accept what cannot be controlled.

3. Learn from experiences in the past. Think about the strength already shown to date to merely survive. Take note about the kinds of skills and strategies that helped in rough times. At this step, acknowledging both positive and negative reactions will be helpful and inform how you wish to respond in the future.

4. Hope. Remain hopeful that the future has yet to be experienced. Things in the past cannot be changed. Anticipate change as a new adventure without the anxiety of the unknown. You embody an un-tapped inner strength to maintain your hope.

5. Actually care for yourself. Seek activities, hobbies, and/or learn new skills that are enjoyable. Practice mindfulness! Think about untried activities as new adventures ripe with opportunities to learn something new.

6. Draw on your power to visualize and create the results you desire. Nothing beats a failure but a try.

ACHIEVING THE GOALS OF WELLNESS WHILE FACING THE UNKNOWN

To be mentally well during chaos in our communities and difficulties in our relationships with others, empowerment is the key. One needs different ideas focused on igniting an epiphany for better living. However, striving for goals is not an easy or straight path. The many twists and turns toward finding one's purpose eventually blossom into a larger journey toward new realities. What this book tried to offer within its pages is a road map toward finding new ways to achieve a more fulfilled and accomplished life.

In the midst of all this, the struggle of keeping depression at bay is to be the hardest fight that one must take. With all these different matters bombarding one's psyche, keeping mentally balanced is worth more now than ever. It is important to take care of each other while dealing with a dozen uncertainties. A major point of this work is to ask our readers to take care of themselves. Having the wherewithal to deal with what is going on in our lives and becoming a mantle of strength is the most relevant thing that a person can do during this time.

IN CONCLUSION . . .

Where do we go from here? Writing this book on depression for African Americans was a journey we all wanted to take and eagerly began. We talked with each other, we debated the finer points on which topics to include and how to share this information with others. Many times we were worried that the messages we wanted to share would not make it past editing. Yet here we are . . . at the end of the book. A dream fulfilled.

As stated in the preface, *African Americans and Depression* was conceived and written to offer information about depression with specific attention to African Americans. Depression is painful, lonely, scary, and can ruin the best life plans. We write about depression because we understand the cultural norms around secrecy and avoidance practices of our people. Our experience in the field, classroom, and with our own research has taught us many lessons about how to approach this topic sensitively and with cultural attention to people who suffer, those who are caregivers, and persons who provide services. Although we live in modern times and many technological advancements have enhanced information gathering, there is something about discussing depression among African Americans that calls for hushed tones. We believe that no one needs to suffer unnecessarily when there are treatment options.

In writing this book, we held on to five goals:

1. To offer some background information about depression among African Americans;
2. To uncover a pathway to seek treatment options by demystifying the process;
3. To share what communities are involved in by way of responses to interventions and programs;
4. To give insight on how to pay for treatment once the decision is made to seek help; and
5. To offer resources for those wishing to learn more, become more informed about treatment experiences, or are just curious about what other options might be available.

When setting this book down, our readers should also be able to understand what is involved in seeking a healthy life. The most powerful thing one can do is *ask for help*. We hope your journey to wellness begins now.

Appendix

Depression Resources for African Americans

One of the conditions of modern living is dealing with the pain and heartbreak of defeat. Barriers block us from progression. Unforgiving people in our lives refuse to understand our position in an important matter. Humiliation and despair loom over unrepentant acts of racism. Let's face it, our lives are filled with the vagaries of the human condition. What is even more, its darkest aspects do not take a day off. Therefore, it helps to have a refuge to find comfort from the sadness and the hopelessness encountered on a daily basis. In fact, discovering an entire community of caring individuals saves lives. Even more importantly, tragedies are stopped in their tracks before grave harm takes hold.

This appendix provides many different avenues for people in search of information about depression and in need of a helping hand. The following listings also reach out to the families and friends of suffering individuals so that they can, too, get aid in troubling times. The resources below represent culturally sensitive pathways toward understanding and hope. Most importantly, African Americans in dire circumstances will find competent and relevant information to gain epiphanies about themselves and others when seeking care. The readings, websites, organizational centers, and telephone numbers are there to give birth to new beginnings and connections while in convalescence. May you find strength, luck, and hope in the resources below.

Take care,
Cecilia M. Hastings

BOOKS

The texts listed below point toward being a sounding board for afflicted persons and their loved ones. Within their pages, the books included go into further explanation of pertinent issues addressing depression and mental health care. Most importantly, the works direct readers toward immediate solutions and much-needed relief.

Boyd-Franklin, Nancy. *Black Families in Therapy: Understanding the African American Experience*. New York: Guilford Press, 2006.

Boyd-Franklin, Nancy, Elizabeth Cleek, Matt Wofsy, and Brian Mundy. *Therapy in the Real World: Effective Treatments for Challenging Problems*. New York: Guilford Press, 2013.

Danquah, Meri Nana-Ama. *Willow Weep for Me: A Black Woman's Journey through Depression, a Memoir*. New York: Norton, 1998.

Davich, Victor N. *8 Minute Meditation: Quiet Your Mind, Change Your Life*. New York: Perigee, 2004.

Farrar-Rosemon, C. J. *How to Get to the Palace from Your Prison: Joseph's 14 Step Program to Overcome Loneliness, Depression, Discrimination, Barrenness and Abuse*. 2008.

Gotlib, Ian H., and Constance L. Hammen. *Handbook of Depression*, 3rd edition. New York: Guilford Press, 2014.

Hampton, Robert L., Thomas P. Gullotta, and Raymond L. Crowel. *Handbook of African American Health*. New York: Guilford Press, 2010.

Head, John. *Black Men and Depression: Saving Our Lives, Healing Our Families and Friends*. New York: Harlem Moon/Broadway Books, 2004.

Head, John. *Black Men and Depression: Understanding and Overcoming Depression in Black Men*. New York: Harlem Moon/Broadway Books, 2005.

hooks, bell. *Killing Rage: Ending Racism*. New York: H. Holt and Company, 1995.

hooks, bell. *Sisters of the Yam: Black Women and Self-Recovery*. Cambridge, MA: South End Press, 2005.

Hoytt, Eleanor H., and Hilary Beard. *Health First! The Black Woman's Wellness Guide*. New York: Smiley Books, 2012.

Jackson, Leslie C., and Beverly Greene. *Psychotherapy with African American Women: Innovations in Psychodynamic Perspectives and Practice*. New York: Guilford Press, 2000.

Johnson, Waldo E. *Social Work with African American Males: Health, Mental Health, and Social Policy*. New York: Oxford University Press, 2010.

Martin, Marilyn, and Mark Moss. *Saving Our Last Nerve: The Black Woman's Path to Mental Health*. Munster, IN: Hilton Publishing, 2002.

Neal-Barnett, Angela M. *Soothe Your Nerves: The Black Woman's Guide to Understanding and Overcoming Anxiety, Panic, and Fear*. New York: Simon & Schuster, 2003.

Schulz, Amy J., and Leith Mullings. *Gender, Race, Class, and Health: Intersectional Approaches*. San Francisco, CA: Jossey-Bass, 2006.

Taylor, Robert Joseph, Linda M. Chatters, and Jeffrey S. Levin. *Religion in the Lives of African Americans: Social, Psychological, and Health Perspectives*. ThousandOaks, CA: Sage Publications, 2004.

Williams, Terrie M. *Black Pain: It Just Looks Like We're Not Hurting*. New York: Scrivener, 2009.

Wright, Bobby E., PhD. "The Psychopathic Racial Personality." In *The Psychopathic Racial Personality and Other Essays*. Chicago: Third World Press, 1984, 1–11.

COMMUNITY SERVICE PROJECTS WITHIN THE
BLACK GREEK SYSTEM

One of the most relevant aspects of the Black Greek System is their generosity and commitment to the community at large. Through recognizing the toughest problems plaguing the society around them, creating projects and programs become an important aspect of the membership experience. In fact, such devotion to the public is part of a national service initiative. Below are examples of dedication to those in need. In turn, the work accomplishes valuable and noteworthy contacts in the start for a new beginning away from the pain of depression.

Zeta Phi Beta Sorority, Incorporated
Project Z-HOPE for Women
With its origin in 1920, the Zeta Phi Beta sorority founded itself on the premise of finer womanhood and the bonds beyond elitism. In this fashion, the organization created Project Z-HOPE to address the most important problems in the African American community. Z-HOPE stands for Zetas Helping Other People Excel. Through their social outreach, the congregation of women created programs that help sustain the well-being of Black people in the continental United States as well as internationally. One area focused upon in their promise to better the world around them is addressing the specific needs of African American women. Therefore, Project Z-HOPE for Women was developed to focus upon depression, domestic abuse, and other challenges faced by females. If you need more information concerning their endeavors, please do visit their web address, http://zphibtdz.org/programs/z-hope-programs.

Delta Sigma Theta Sorority, Incorporated, and National Black Nurses Association. The National Campaign on Clinical Depression
In acknowledgment of the need to increase awareness within the African American female community, Delta Sigma Theta Sorority, Inc., and the National Black Nurses Association have partnered in the National Campaign on Clinical Depression. You can call their hotline toll-free at 1-(800)-228-1114 for information on support groups and other resources.

MAGAZINE ARTICLES

Here are some worthwhile articles discussing specific issues experienced during the struggle for wellness. The citations tackle the stigma and perception of African Americans diagnosed with depression. The items brought forth also specifically address how the cultural experiences of the African

American community intersect with the pursuit of finding competent care while in the throes of mental illness. Most relevantly, the citations describe candidly the needed empowerment and respect during the process of seeking help.

Hamm, Nia. "Black Folks and Mental Health: Why Do We Suffer in Silence?" *Ebony*, October 1, 2012. Accessed August 20, 2014. http://www.ebony.com/wellness-empowerment/black-folks-and-mental-health-610/2#axzz3HUj8KIOc.
Payne, January W. "Black and Blue: Depression among African-Americans." *US News*, January 16, 2008. Accessed August 20, 2014. http://health.usnews.com/health-news/articles/2008/01/16/black-and-blue-depression-among-african-americans.
Pickens, Josie. "Depression and the Black Superwoman Syndrome." *Ebony*, April 15, 2014. Accessed August 20, 2014. http://www.ebony.com/wellness-empowerment/depression-and-the-black-superwoman-syndrome-777#axzz3HUj8KIOc.
Silverstein, Jason. "How Racism Is Bad for Our Bodies." *Atlantic*, March 12, 2013. Accessed August 20, 2014. http://www.theatlantic.com/health/archive/2013/03/how-racism-is-bad-for-our-bodies/273911.

NEWSPAPER AND BLOG ARTICLES

Using highly accessed and widely read periodicals by the public at large, each article tackles the underlying problems in the African American community when seeking help for depression. Pointedly, the works especially attack the problems experienced in fighting the negativity against those trying to make sense out of their troubled lives. The subject matter addressed in this portion of the resources works toward ending the silence around mental health issues.

Bahrampour, Tara. "Therapists Say African Americans Are Increasingly Seeking Help for Mental Illness." *Washington Post*, July 9, 2013. Accessed August 21, 2014. http://www.washingtonpost.com/local/therapists-say-african-americans-are-increasingly-seeking-help-for-mental-illness/2013/07/09/9b15cb4c-e400-11e2-a11e-c2ea876a8f30_story.html.
Coleman, Monica A. "Four Black Church Resources That Can Help People Living with Depression." *The Blog (The Huffington Post)*, July 1, 2014. Accessed August 21, 2014. http://www.huffingtonpost.com/monica-a-coleman/4-black-church-resources-_b_5547414.html.
Edmonds, Heather. "African Americans and Mental Illness: 'It's Not Just the Blues.'" *Ideas and Insights Blog*, May 3, 2011. Accessed August 21, 2014. http://www.iqsolutions.com/ideas-and-insights/blog/african-americans-mental-illness-its-not-just-blues.
Norwood, Kimberly. "Why I Fear for My Sons." *CNN Opinion*, August 25, 2014. Accessed August 25, 2014. http://us.cnn.com/2014/08/25/opinion/norwood-ferguson-sons-brown-police/index.html?c=page=3.
Sanders, Joshunda. "Mainstream Media Tend to Ignore Blacks' Mental Health Problems." *Maynard Media Center on Structural Inequity*, July 11, 2012. Accessed August 21, 2014. http://mije.org/mmcsi/health/mainstream-media-tend-ignore-blacks%E2%80%99-mental-health-problems.
Talbert, Marcia Wade. "Challenging the Stigma of Mental Illness." *Black Enterprise*, January 8, 2015. Accessed August 21, 2014. http://www.blackenterprise.com/news/challenging-the-stigma-of-mental-illness/.
Valleskey, Brianna. "Depression and Suicide in African Americans: Symptoms and Getting Help." *BLAC Detroit*, July 2012. Accessed August 20, 2014. http://www.blacdetroit.com/

BLAC-Detroit/July-2012/Depression-and-Suicide-in-African-Americans-Symptoms-and-Getting-Help/.

ORGANIZATIONS

While undergoing the symptoms of depression, mental health associations play a key role providing help for persons with nowhere else to turn. The following large groups battle the various aspects of depression, domestic violence, and the silence around mental illness stigma. The organizations exist because they work in the trenches every day of the year. Please do look below and visit the various sites to gain strength and hope.

African American Family Services (AAFS) https://www.facebook.com/pages/African-American-Family-Services/143304565712680
With its goal toward finding assistance applicable to Black culture, African American Family Services flourished into a place striving for the utmost healing of its clients. Since 1975, it has tackled domestic abuse, suicide, and depression. Working with the Black family, the center tries to prevent situations associated with violence.

AfricanAmericanTherapists.com   http://africanamericantherapists.com/#sthash.0SfAAVtN.dpbs
This organization is a psychiatric outreach service so that communities of color can find mental health practitioners suitable for their health care needs. The site especially has a well-filled directory to guide a user toward appropriate resources.

Black Mental Health Alliance (BMHA) http://blackmentalhealth.com/index.html
The Black Mental Health Alliance gears its energies toward therapeutic intervention via consultation, group meetings, and providing appropriate information to its clientele. The organization has worked on alleviating mental distress in the African American community through its belief of spiritual renewal and strong support since its beginning in 1984. Ultimately, the consortium of board participants hopes to enable a welcoming place in which shame and loneliness can be eliminated through nurturing and respectful service.

The Black Mind http://media-garden.org/theblackmind/about.html
With the goal of breaking down aspects of fear associated with mental health, the group formed in 2012 in order to exchange ideas and become a think tank for helping the African American community reach the goals of significant wellness. Headed by a board, one of the main practices of the

organization is to not let one suffer in silence and to share his or her experience with others.

Mental Health America (MHA) http://www.mentalhealthamerica.net
Beginning in 1909, this group and its countrywide affiliates yearn to educate, advocate, and bring mental health resources to diverse communities.

National Alliance on Mental Illness (NAMI) http://www.nami.org/
Starting in 2002, this site pools information for aiding people of color. Secondly, it coordinates resources and places so that persons in cultural and racial communities can seek terms of assistance. It works to end discriminatory practices in mental health.

Samaritan Behavioral Health (SBH) http://www.sbhihelp.org/html/AfAmDepression.htm
This is an organization in Ohio that pays attention to mental health services regarding people of color. It especially focuses on crisis situations.

Substance Abuse and Mental Health Services Administration (SAMHSA) http://www.samhsa.gov/
Ensconced within the Department of Human Health and Services, this agency works on establishing mental and active wellness within the United States. Initiated by Congress in 1992, the center works on eliminating the factors that tear at the seams of the national fabric, such as alcohol and drugs. One of its main goals is to help communities of color heal and work toward betterment. "Stories That Heal" is one such program targeted at African Americans.

PDF INFORMATION

The authors commit to using emerging digital media in the fight against depression. In similar fashion, the following listings offer lengthy readings that provide references to more extensive services a person can consult on their path to wellness. The files offer a total buffet of choices to find help and information. What is especially great is that the readings are portable and can fit within the apps on one's electronic device.

California Reducing Disparities Project and Strategic Planning Workgroup. *African American Mental Health Providers Directory for California Residents*. African American Health Institute, May 2012. Accessed August 20, 2014. http://www.aahi-sbc.org/uploads/African_Am_CRDP_MHDirectoryFINAL.pdf.
Centers for Disease Control and Prevention, Substance Abuse and Mental Health Services Administration, National Association of County Behavioral Health & Developmental Dis-

ability Directors, National Institute of Mental Health, The Carter Center Mental Health Program. *Attitudes toward Mental Illness: Results from the Behavior Risk Factor Surveillance System.* Atlanta, GA: Centers for Disease Control and Prevention, 2012. Accessed August 21, 2014. http://www.cdc.gov/hrqol/mental_health_reports/pdf/brfss_report_insidepages.pdf.

Mental Health Association. "Clinical Depression in African Americans." Accessed August 18, 2014. http://www.mhacolorado.org/file_depot/0-10000000/30000-40000/31946/folder/76278/Depression and African Americans.pdf

NAMI. The African American Community Mental Health Fact Sheet. Accessed August 18, 2014. http://www.nami.org/Template.cfm?Section=Fact_Sheets&Template=/Management/ContentDisplay.cfm&ContentID=88872.

NAMI. A Family Guide—Choosing the Right Treatment: What Families Need to Know About Evidence-Based Practices. Accessed August 18, 2014. http://www.nami.org/Content/ContentGroups/CAAC/ChoosingRightTreatment.pdf.

National Alliance on Mental Illness. "African American Women and Depression Fact Sheet." Accessed August 18, 2014. http://www.nami.org/Content/NavigationMenu/Mental_Illnesses/Women_and_Depression/african_american_women.pdf.

The Center for African American Health. "Depression and African Americans." Accessed August 18, 2014. http://www.caahealth.org/repository/files/pdf/Depression%26AfricanAmer.pdf.

U.S. Department of Health and Human Services, Office on Women's Health, 2009. *Action Steps for Improving Women's Mental Health.* Washington, DC: U.S. Department of Health and Human Services, Office on Women's Health. Accessed October 28, 2014. http://www.dhcs.ca.gov/services/owh/Documents2/Articles/MentalHealthActionSteps.pdf.

U.S. Department of Health and Human Services, Office of Women's Health, 2009. *Women's Mental Health: What It Means to You.* Washington, DC: U.S. Department of Health and Human Services, Office on Women's Health. Accessed October 28, 2014. https://store.samhsa.gov/shin/content/OWH09-CONSUMER/OWH09-CONSUMER.pdf.

PSYCHOLOGICAL HELP CENTERS

Psychological Help Centers are there for persons who need to find an immediate resource on the Internet. Accessing these pages leads to information on finding localized and affiliated sites within one's hometown. The citations below often have advice on getting critical care while experiencing dire situations.

California Black Women's Health Project (CBWHP). http://www.cabwhp.org/. Accessed August 20, 2014.

Originating in a partnership with the UCLA Self-Help Center, CBWHP works to provide resources for African American women in the throes of mental illness. Going strong after sixteen years, the center reaches out through its strongest asset: to provide advocacy in order to knock down social disparities in mental health services.

The Center for African American Health.http://www.caahealth.org/. Accessed August 18, 2014.

Started in Denver, Colorado, it is a base of operations for aiding the African American community in terms of mental health and well-being. The site educates its constituency on helping themselves to achieve success in eliminating their issues and conquering disparities within the therapeutic realm. Integrating the tradition of religion within Black culture, it strives to enable its members to take command of their own destiny through faith and spirituality.

Kristin Brooks Hope Center http://www.hopeline.com/

People in crisis generally don't have the energy or ability to take on a long search for help. The mission has been to offer *hope* and the option to *live* to those in the deepest emotional pain. Those looking for support dial 1-800-SUICIDE and are seamlessly connected to an available certified crisis center nearest to the calling location.

SCHOLARLY LITERATURE

The search for wellness also involves finding sources within academia from various experts specialized in their field of study. Consulting their sources can point toward new ways to perceive the impact of depression. Furthermore, reading the texts might inspire the person diagnosed with depression to approach the illness in an alternative way. Thus, the subsequent citations are presented in such a manner to elicit reflective thoughts about how to deal with such a difficult disease.

Akbar, Na'Im. "Africentric Social Sciences for Human Liberation." *Journal of Black Studies* 14, no. 4 (1984): 395–414.

Baldwin, J. A. "African (Black) Psychology: Issues and Synthesis." *Journal of Black Studies* 16, no. 3 (1986): 235–49.

Carruthers, Jacob. "Towards the Development of a Black Social Theory." In *Howard University Graduate Student Council's Distinguished Lecture Series*. Washington, DC, 1989.

Cunningham, Phillippe B., Sharon L. Foster, and Sarah E. Warner. "Culturally Relevant Family-Based Treatment for Adolescent Delinquency and Substance Abuse: Understanding Within-Session Processes." *Journal of Clinical Psychology* 66, no. 8 (2010): 830–46.

Davis, S. K., A. D. Williams, and M. Akinyela. "An Afrocentric Approach to Building Cultural Relevance in Social Work Research." *Journal of Black Studies* 41, no. 2 (2010): 1–13.

Gilbert, D. J., A. R. Harvey, and F. Z. Belgrave. "Advancing the Afrocentric Paradigm Shift Discourse: Building toward Evidence-Based Afrocentric Interventions in Social Work Practice with African Americans." *Social Work* 54, no. 3 (2009): 243–52.

Harvey, Aminifu R., and Robert B. Hill. "Afrocentric Youth and Family Rites of Passage Program: Promoting Resilience among At-Risk African American Youths." *Social Work* 49, no. 1 (2004): 65–74.

Helms, Janet E. "An Update of Helms's White and People of Color Racial Identity Models." In *Handbook of Multicultural Counseling*, ed. Joseph G. Ponterotto et al. Thousand Oaks, CA: Sage Publications, 1995.

Nobles, Wade W. "African Consciousness and Liberation Struggles: Implications for the Development and Construction of Scientific Paradigms." In *Fanon Research and Development Conference*. Port of Spain, Trinidad, 1978.

Nobles, Wade W. "African Philosophy: Foundation for Black Psychology." In *Black Psychology*, ed. Reginald L. Jones. Berkeley, CA: Cobb & Henry, 1991.

Phinney, Jean S. "When We Talk About American Ethnic Groups, What Do We Mean?" *American Psychologist* 51, no. 9 (1996): 918–27.

Sherr, Michael F. "The Afrocentric Paradigm: A Pragmatic Discourse about Social Work Practice with African Americans." *Journal of Human Behavior in the Social Environment* 13, no. 3 (2006): 1–17.

WEBSITES

The Internet has left an indelible mark on communications within three decades. Since its birth in the late twentieth century, the World Wide Web has been a place for people to exchange ideas, bond, and seek new forms of information. Online, like-minded people seek someone else to talk to and listen to. Websites have been an integral part of the structure of the Internet. Numerous places on the Internet carry a plethora of information to unite disparate people under one subject. This is what the following sources do when people diagnosed with depression look for help online. The websites are there to offer visitors substantial ways to work toward recovery via directories, helpful newsletters, and personal intervention.

African-American Mental Health Providers Directory http://aamhp.com/

This website exists as a resource in the search for African Americans involved in the psychological and social welfare field. The compendium especially deals with marriage and family therapeutic services. It also lists fare for its associated groups and organizations as further areas of help and education.

American Foundation for Suicide Prevention http://www.afsp.org/

When loved ones are on the brink of despair, this online place exists as an immediate panacea. The American Foundation for Suicide Prevention works diligently to conduct research and provide resources in order to combat suicide. Not only does it have a national presence, local chapters exist as well. One of the most important things the website does is to give a voice to the pain sufferers feel while on the road to getting better.

American Psychiatric Association. "African Americans." http://www.psychiatry.org/african-americans

With a robust membership of more than 35,000, the American Psychiatric Association advocates for exceptional mental health care in America for persons afflicted with mental illness. The organization also advocates for the respect, dignity, and well-being of the patients and families within the realm of medicine. This is especially the case for African Americans. On its site, it is well noted that African Americans with mental illness need to be recognized and treated with quality by professionals within the psychiatry discipline. Therefore, the page outlines several ways communities of color can access much-needed support and relief while dealing with depression.

BlackCounselors.com http://www.blackcounselors.com/

Black Counselors helps people find the African American therapists, psychologists, psychiatrists, marriage and family counselors, social workers, and licensed professional counselors listed on their directory and provides their license or certification information, which is available for verification through their state's regulating body.

Black Mental Health Alliance (BMHA) http://blackmentalhealth.com/

Working on erasing the stigma mental illness has in the African American community, the Black Mental Health Alliance takes a holistic approach in its advocacy. Since the group's inception in 1984, they have especially strived to create programs, sponsor events, and disseminate educational resources to help the public understand the serious impact depression and its ilk possesses. One of their greatest goals is for communities of color to receive the utmost care while experiencing psychological issues.

BlackMentalHealthNet.com (BMHN) http://www.blackmentalhealthnet.com/

Using the full benefits of social media and the World Wide Web, BMHN reaches out to the African American community as a sanctuary for those affected by mental illness. Forums, newsletters, and videos contribute to breaking down the stress and fear related to crisis situations. The site's strongest goal is to stop the isolation that Black people have when dealing with psychological and familial distress. What is truly emphasized is the ability to break the silence and speak out.

BlackWomenHealth (BWH) http://www.blackwomenshealth.com/

This site works to educate and enlighten Black women on methods to take better care of themselves. Although the organization discusses many medical issues, there is a section dealing with mental illness. With the main focus on clinical depression, the web page contains a plethora of culturally sensitive information so that women of color can find what they need to embark on working to eliminate their mental illness.

Center for Advancing Health (CFAH) http://www.cfah.org/

The Center for Advancing Health helps patients become more vocal in treatment issues. The site uses educational resources to enlighten its visitors to make wise choices in health care. Finding a voice while in recovery, the patient can gain more self-esteem and confidence in getting the best care possible. Therefore, these terms solidify CFAH's motto of "patient engagement."

Community Tool Box http://ctb.dept.ku.edu/en/table-of-contents
The Community Tool Box is designed to inform families about evidence-based practices (EBPs) in children's mental health and to share information on an array of treatment and support options.

The Kaiser Permanente Center for Health Research Download Site for Youth Depression Treatment and Prevention Programs http://www.kpchr.org/research/public/acwd/acwd.html
These materials are for the use of mental health professionals to deliver group cognitive behavioral treatment or prevention to teenagers. These are not self-help materials for the direct use of depressed teenagers and their families.

Lee   Thompson   Young   Foundation   http://www.leethompsonyoungfoundation.org/
Named after the actor who tragically took his life in 2013, this online resource focuses on the mental health concerns of those afflicted with feelings of depression, suicide, and other aspects of crisis. Most importantly, the organization emphasizes culturally sensitive help to bring about a restoration of wellness. Its main goal is to erase the negative connotation that psychological distress may bring.

National Alliance on Mental Illness. NAMI Multicultural Action Center http://www.nami.org/Template.cfm?section=multicultural_support
One of the premiere sites fighting the ravages of mental illness, the National Alliance on Mental Illness works to educate its visitors on how to recognize the signs of clinical depression. One special aspect of its endeavors is to help communities of color become more adept in coping skills while dealing with this terrible disease.

National Organization for People of Color against Suicide (NOPCAS) http://nopcas.com/
Dedicated to preventing suicide in communities of color nationally, NOPCAS works on intervention before the tragedy strikes. Prevention and awareness become the main themes of educating the public. The Internet is strongly used for this purpose because of its wide reach. The organization especially provides opportunities to reach out to clinicians in the mental health discipline to address the unique needs of patients of color. The devastation of

remaining silent because of stigma is taken head-on so that suffering from depression does not remain hidden from view. What it comes down to is that the needs of cultures of color will not be ignored.

Substance Abuse and Mental Health Services Administration (SAMHSA) http://www.samhsa.gov/
    Connected to the nationwide organization, this site focuses on working to educate African Americans as well as other communities of color in mental wellness. Articles and other educational resources also provide information tailored to the needs of its audience.

Bibliography

Agyemang, A. A., B. Mezuk, P. Perrin, and B. Rybarczyk. "Quality of Depression Treatment in Black Americans with Major Depression and Comorbid Medical Illness." *General Hospital Psychiatry* 36, no. 4 (July–August 2014): 431–36.

Akbar, Na'Im. "Africentric Social Sciences for Human Liberation." *Journal of Black Studies* 14, no. 4 (1984): 395–414.

———. "The Evolution of Human Psychology for African Americans." In *Black Psychology*, edited by Reginald L. Jones. Berkeley, CA: Cobb & Henry, 1991.

American Psychiatric Association, ed. *Diagnostic and Statistical Manual of Mental Disorders (DSM-V)*. 5th edition. Arlington, VA: American Psychiatric Publishing, 2013.

American Psychological Association. *APA Dictionary of Psychology*. Washington, DC: American Psychological Association, 2007.

Andrews, Dale P. *Practical Theology for Black Churches: Bridging Black Theology and African American Folk Religion* [in English]. Louisville, KY: Westminster John Knox Press, 2002.

Arunkumar, Revathy, Carol Midgley, and Tim Urdan. "Perceiving High or Low Home-School Dissonance: Longitudinal Effects on Adolescent Emotional and Academic Well-Being." *Journal of Research on Adolescence* 9, no. 4 (1999): 441–66.

Assari, S. "Chronic Medical Conditions and Major Depressive Disorder: Differential Role of Positive Religious Coping among African Americans, Caribbean Blacks and Non-Hispanic Whites." *International Journal of Preventative Medicine* 5, no. 4 (April 2014): 405–13.

Atkins, Marc S., Kimberly E. Hoagwood, Krista Kutash, and Edward Seidman. "Toward the Integration of Education and Mental Health in Schools." *Administration and Policy in Mental Health and Mental Health Services Research* 37, no. 1–2 (2010): 40–47.

Bailey, Martha J., and Sheldon Danziger, eds. *Legacies of the War on Poverty*, The National Poverty Center Series on Poverty and Public Policy. New York: Russell Sage Foundation, 2013.

Bambara, Toni Cade. *The Salt Eaters* [in English]. New York: Random House, 1980.

Beeghly, Marjorie, Karen L. Olson, M. Katherine Weinberg, Snaltze Charlot Pierre, Nikora Downey, and Edward Z. Tronick. "Prevalence, Stability, and Socio-Demographic Correlates of Depressive Symptoms in Black Mothers During the First 18 Months Postpartum." *Maternal and Child Health Journal* 7, no. 3 (2003): 157–68.

Billingsley, Andrew. *Mighty Like a River: The Black Church and Social Reform* [in English]. New York: Oxford University Press, 1999.

Borchard, Therese J. "6 Steps for Beating Depression." http://psychcentral.com/blog/archives/2009/07/09/6-steps-for-beating-depression/.

Boutin-Foster, Carla, Ebony Scott, Jennifer Melendez, Anna Rodriguez, Rosio Ramos, Bala-venkatesh Kanna, and Walid Michelen. "Ethical Considerations for Conducting Health Disparities Research in Community Health Centers: A Social-Ecological Perspective." *American Journal of Public Health* 103, no. 12 (2013): 2179–84.

Bowie, S. L., and D. M. Dopwell. "Metastressors as Barriers to Self-Sufficiency among TANF-Reliant African American and Latina Women." *Affilia: Journal of Women and Social Work* 28, no. 2 (2013): 177–93.

Boyd-Franklin, Nancy. "Incorporating Spirituality and Religion into the Treatment of African American Clients." *Counseling Psychologist* 38, no. 7 (2010): 976–1000.

Boyd-Franklin, Nancy. "Recurrent Themes in the Treatment of African American Women in Group Therapy." *Women & Therapy* 11 (2003): 25–40.

Boyd-Franklin, Nancy, Elizabeth Cleek, Matt Wofsy, and Brian Mundy. *Therapy in the Real World: Effective Treatments for Challenging Problems*. New York: Guilford Press, 2013.

Boykin, A. Wade, and Forrest D. Toms. "Black Child Socialization: A Conceptual Framework." In *Black Children: Social, Educational, and Parental Environments*, edited by Harriette Pipes McAdoo and John Lewis McAdoo, 33–52. Beverly Hills: Sage Publications, 1985.

Breslau, Joshua, Kenneth S. Kendler, Maxwell Su, Sergio Gaxiola-Aguilar, and Ronald C. Kessler. "Lifetime Risk and Persistence of Psychiatric Disorders across Ethnic Groups in the United States." *Psychological Medicine* 35, no. 3 (2005): 317–27.

Bronfenbrenner, Urie. "Contexts of Child Rearing: Problems and Prospects." *American Psychologist* 34, no. 10 (1979): 844–50.

———. *Making Human Beings Human: Bioecological Perspectives on Human Development*. Newbury Park, CA: Sage, 2005.

Brook, Judith S., Martin Whiteman, Carolyn Nomura, Ann Scovell Gordon, and Patricia Cohen. "Personality, Family, and Ecological Influences on Adolescent Drug Use: A Developmental Analysis." *Journal of Chemical Dependency Treatment* 1, no. 2 (1988): 123–61.

Carruthers, Jacob. "Towards the Development of a Black Social Theory." In *Howard University Graduate Student Council's Distinguished Lecture Series*. Washington, DC, 1989.

Carter Center. "The President's New Freedom Commission on Mental Health: Transforming the Vision." In *The Nineteenth Annual Rosalynn Carter Symposium on Mental Health Policy*, 2003.

Census, U.S. Bureau of the. "Current Population." http://www.census.gov.

Center for Behavioral Health Statistics and Quality. "Results from the 2012 National Survey on Drug Use and Health: Summary of National Findings." Rockville, MD: Substance Abuse and Mental Health Services Administration, 2013.

Centers for Disease Control and Prevention. "Depression in the U.S. Household Population, 2009–2012." http://www.cdc.gov/nchs/pressroom/upcoming.htm.

———. "Minority Health: Black or African Americans." http://www.cdc.gov/minorityhealth/populations/remp/black.html.

Centers for Medicare & Medicaid Services. "Children's Health Insurance Program."http://www.cms.gov/Outreach-and-Education/American-Indian-Alaska-Native/AIAN/CHIP-Grantees/Overview.html.

———. "Medicaid.gov: Keeping America Healthy."http://www.medicaid.gov/.

———. "Medicare." http://www.cms.gov/Medicare/Medicare.html.

———. "The Mental Health Parity and Addiction Equity Act." http://www.cms.gov/CCIIO/Programs-and-Initiatives/Other-Insurance-Protections/mhpaea_factsheet.html.

Choi, N. G., and J. M. Gonzalez. "Geriatric Mental Health Clinicians' Perceptions of Barriers and Contributors to Retention of Older Minorities in Treatment: An Exploratory Study." *Clinical Gerontologist* 28, no. 3 (2005): 3–25.

Claxton, Gary, Matthew Rae, Nirmita Panchal, Janet Lundy, and Anthony Damico. "Employer Health Benefits: 2011 Annual Survey." Edited by The Kaiser Family Foundation, 2011.

Claxton, Gary, Matthew Rae, Nirmita Panchal, Heidi Whitmore, Anthony Damico, and Kevin Kenward. "Health Benefits in 2014: Stability in Premiums and Coverage for Employer-Sponsored Plans." *Health Affairs* 33, no. 10 (October 1, 2014): 1851–60.

Crockett, Kathy, Caron Zlotnick, Melvin Davis, Nanetta Payne, and Rosie Washington. "A Depression Preventive Intervention for Rural Low-Income African-American Pregnant Women at Risk for Postpartum Depression." *Archives of Women's Mental Health* 11, no. 5–6 (2008): 319–25.

Cunningham, Phillippe B., Sharon L. Foster, and Sarah E. Warner. "Culturally Relevant Family-Based Treatment for Adolescent Delinquency and Substance Abuse: Understanding Within-Session Processes." *Journal of Clinical Psychology* 66, no. 8 (August 2010): 830–46.

Davis, Robert. "Suicide among Young Blacks: Trends and Perspectives." *Phylon (1960)* 41, no. 3 (1980): 223–29.

DeNavas-Walt, Carmen, Bernadette D. Proctor, and Jessica C. Smith. "Income, Poverty, and Health Insurance Coverage in the United States: 2010." Edited by U.S. Census Bureau, 87. Washington, DC: U.S. Government Printing Office, 2011.

Garibaldi, Antoine M. "Educating and Motivating African American Males to Succeed." *The Journal of Negro Education* 61, no. 1 (1992): 4–11.

Gilbert, D. J., A. R. Harvey, and F. Z. Belgrave. "Advancing the Africentric Paradigm Shift Discourse: Building toward Evidence-Based Africentric Interventions in Social Work Practice with African Americans." *Social Work* 54, no. 3 (July 2009): 243–52.

Gonzalez, H. M., W. A. Vega, D. R. Williams, W. Tarraf, B. T. West, and H. W. Neighbors. "Depression Care in the United States: Too Little for Too Few." *Archives of General Psychiatry* 67, no. 1 (January 2010): 37–46.

Gotlib, Ian H., and Constance L. Hammen, eds. *Handbook of Depression*. 3rd edition. New York: Guilford Press, 2014.

Greenberg, Paul E., Ronald C. Kessler, Howard G. Birnbaum, Stephanie A. Leong, Sarah W. Lowe, Patricia A. Berglund, and Patricia K. Corey-Lisle. "The Economic Burden of Depression in the United States: How Did It Change between 1990 and 2000?" *Journal of Clinical Psychiatry* 64, no. 12 (2003): 1465–74.

Greene, Beverly. "Psychotherapy with African American Women: Integrating Feminist and Psychodynamic Models." *Smith College Studies in Social Work* 67, no. 3 (1997): 299–322.

Griffith, D. M., J. L. Johnson, R. Zhang, H. W. Neighbors, and J. S. Jackson. "Ethnicity, Nativity, and the Health of American Blacks." *Journal of Health Care for the Poor and Underserved* 22, no. 1 (February 2011): 142–56.

Gutierrez, Lorraine M. "Working with Women of Color: An Empowerment Perspective." *Social Work* 35, no. 2 (1990): 149–53.

Hamm, Nia. "Black Folks and Mental Health: Why Do We Suffer in Silence?" *Ebony*, October 1, 2012.

Harvey, Aminifu R., and Robert B. Hill. "Africentric Youth and Family Rites of Passage Program: Promoting Resilience among At-Risk African American Youths." *Social Work* 49, no. 1 (2004): 65–74.

Hastings, Julia F. "Understanding Diabetes and Depression among African Americans in California and New York." California and New York: National Institute on Minority Health and Health Disparities (NIMHD), 2014.

Head, John. *Black Men and Depression: Understanding and Overcoming Depression in Black Men*. New York: Harlem Moon/Broadway Books, 2005.

———. *Black Men and Depression: Saving Our Lives, Healing Our Families and Friends*. Crown Publishing Group, 2010.

Helms, Janet E. "An Update of Helms's White and People of Color Racial Identity Models." In *Handbook of Multicultural Counseling*, edited by Joseph G. Ponterotto et al. Thousand Oaks, CA: Sage Publications, 1995.

Hendrickson, Jo M., Carl R. Smith, Alan R. Frank, and Cheryl Merical. "Decision Making Factors Associated with Placement of Students with Emotional and Behavioral Disorders in Restrictive Educational Settings." *Education and Treatment of Children* 21, no. 3 (1998): 275–302.

Herbeck, D. M., J. C. West, I. Ruditis, F. F. Duffy, D. J. Fitek, C. C. Bell, and Lonnie R. Snowden. "Variations in Use of Second Generation Antipsychotic Medication by Race among Adult Psychiatric Patients." *Psychiatric Services* 55 (2004): 677–84.

Hoffman, Catherine, and A. Schlobohm. *The Kaiser Commission on Medicaid and the Uninsured: Chart Book*, 2nd edition. Washington, DC: Henry J. Kaiser Foundation, 2000.

Holahan, John, and Alshadye Yemane. "Enrollment Is Driving Medicaid Costs—but Two Targets Can Yield Savings." *Health Affairs* 28, no. 5 (2009): 1453–65.

hooks, bell. *Sisters of the Yam: Black Women and Self-Recovery*. Cambridge, MA: South End Press, 2005.

Hopps, June G., and Elaine Pinderhughes. *Group Work with Overwhelmed Clients: How the Power of Groups Can Help People Transform Their Lives* [in English]. New York: Free Press, 1999.

Hosp, John L., and Daniel J. Reschly. "Disproportionate Representation of Minority Students in Special Education: Academic, Demographic, and Economic Predictors." *Exceptional Children* 70, no. 2 (2004): 185–99.

House Committee on Ways and Means. "Green Book." Washington, D.C.: GPO, 2008.

———. "Green Book." Washington, D.C.: GPO, 2012.

Hoytt, Eleanor H., and Hilary Beard. *Health First!: The Black Woman's Wellness Guide*. New York: Smiley Books, 2012.

Hudson, D. L., H. W. Neighbors, A. T. Geronimus, and J. S. Jackson. "The Relationship between Socioeconomic Position and Depression among a US Nationally Representative Sample of African Americans." *Social Psychiatry in Epidemiology* 47, no. 3 (March 2012): 373–81.

Hughes, Jan, and Oi-man Kwok. "Influence of Student-Teacher and Parent-Teacher Relationships on Lower Achieving Readers' Engagement and Achievement in the Primary Grades." *Journal of Educational Psychology* 99, no. 1 (2007): 39–51.

Husband, Charles. "Recognising Diversity and Developing Skills: The Proper Role of Transcultural Communication." *European Journal of Social Work* 3, no. 3 (2000): 225–34.

Institute of Medicine. "Emergency Medical Services at the Crossroads." Washington, DC, 2007.

———. *Unequal Treatment: Confronting Racial and Ethnic Disparities in Health Care*. Edited by Institute of Medicine. Washington, DC: The National Academies Press, 2002.

Jackson, James S., Cleopatra Howard Caldwell, and Sherrill L. Sellers, eds. *Researching Black Communities: A Methodological Guide*. Ann Arbor, MI: The University of Michigan Press, 2012.

Jackson, James S., M. Torres, Cleo H. Caldwell, Harold W. Neighbors, Randy Nesse, Robert Joseph Taylor, Steve J. Trierweiler, and David R. Williams. "The National Survey of American Life: A Study of Racial, Ethnic, and Cultural Influences on Mental Disorders and Mental Health." *International Journal of Methods in Psychiatric Research* 13 (2004): 196–207.

Jackson, Leslie C., and Beverly Greene. "Review of Psychotherapy with African American Women: Innovations in Psychodynamic Perspectives and Practices." *The Psychoanalytic Quarterly* 72 (2003): 524–26.

James, Sherman A. "John Henryism and the Health of African Americans." *Culture, Medicine and Psychiatry* 18 (1994): 163–82.

Joe, Sean. "Implications of Focusing on Black Youth Self-Destructive Behaviors Instead of Suicide When Designing Preventative Interventions." In *Reducing Adolescent Risk: Toward an Integrated Approach*, edited by Daniel Romer, 325–32. Thousand Oaks, CA: Sage Publications, 2003.

———. "Implications of National Suicide Trends for Social Work Practice with Black Youth." *Child and Adolescent Social Work Journal* 23, no. 4 (2006): 458–71.

———. "Suicide among African Americans: A Male's Burden." In *Social Work with African American Males: Health, Mental Health, and Social Policy*, edited by Waldo E. Johnson, 243–62. New York: Oxford University Press, 2010.

Joe, Sean, and Mark S. Kaplan. "Firearm-Related Suicide among Young African-American Males." *Psychiatric Services* 53, no. 3 (2002): 332–34.

Jones, Lani V., and Briggett Ford. "Depression in African American Women: Application of a Psychosocial Competence Practice Framework." *Affilia* 23, no. 2 (2008): 134–43.

Jones, Lani V., Laura Hopson, Lynn Warner, Eric R. Hardiman, and Tana James. "A Qualitative Study of Black Women's Experiences in Drug Abuse and Mental Health Services." *Affilia* (2014).

Kaiser Commission on Medicaid and the Uninsured. "Fact Sheet, Health Coverage by Race and Ethnicity: The Potential Impact of the Affordable Care Act Executive Summary."http://kaiserfamilyfoundation.files.wordpress.com/2014/07/8423-health-coverage-by-race-and-ethnicity.pdf.

Kane, Robert, Rosalie Kane, Neva Kaye, Robert Mollica, Trish Riley, Paul Saucier, Kimberly Irvin Snow, and Louise Starr. "The Basics of Managed Care." In *Managed Care: Handbook for the Aging Network*, edited by Robert Kane and Louise Starr, 219. Minneapolis, MN: National LTC Resource Center, 1996.

Kolko, David J., Michael S. Hurlburt, Jinjin Zhang, Richard P. Barth, Laurel K. Leslie, and Barbara J. Burns. "Posttraumatic Stress Symptoms in Children and Adolescents Referred for Child Welfare Investigation: A National Sample of In-Home and Out-of-Home Care." *Child Maltreatment* 15, no. 1 (2010): 48–63.

Kubrin, Charis E., and Tim Wadsworth. "Explaining Suicide among Blacks and Whites: How Socioeconomic Factors and Gun Availability Affect Race-Specific Suicide Rates." *Social Science Quarterly* 90, no. 5 (2009): 1203–27.

Kunen, Seth, Ronda Niederhauser, Patrick O. Smith, Jerry A. Morris, and Brian D. Marx. "Race Disparities in Psychiatric Rates in Emergency Departments." *Journal of Consulting and Clinical Psychology* 73, no. 1 (2005): 116–26.

Ladner, Joyce A. "Introduction to Tomorrow's Tomorrow: The Black Woman." In *Feminism & Methodology*, edited by Sandra Harding, 74–83. Bloomington, IN: Indiana University Press, 1987.

Lee, Carol D. "Cultural Modeling: CHAT as a Lens for Understanding Instructional Discourse Based on African American English Discourse Patterns." In *Vygotsky's Educational Theory in Cultural Context*, edited by Alex Kozulin et al., 393–410. New York: Cambridge University Press, 2003.

———. "Is October Brown Chinese? A Cultural Modeling Activity System for Underachieving Students." *American Educational Research Journal* 38, no. 1 (2001): 97–141.

Lincoln, C. Eric, and Lawrence H. Mamiya. *The Black Church in the African-American Experience* [in English]. Durham: Duke University Press, 1990.

Lindsey, Kenneth P., and Gordon L. Paul. "Involuntary Commitments to Public Mental Illness Issues Involving the Overrepresentation of and Assessment of Relevant Functioning." *Psychological Bulletin* 106, no. 2 (1989): 171–83.

Lynn, Marvin. "Race, Culture, and the Education of African Americans." *Educational Theory* 56, no. 1 (2006): 107–19.

Martin, L. A., H. W. Neighbors, and D. M. Griffith. "The Experience of Symptoms of Depression in Men vs. Women: Analysis of the National Comorbidity Survey Replication." *JAMA Psychiatry* 70, no. 10 (October 2013): 1100–6.

Martin, Pamela. "Theology and Faith Development among African American Adolescents: An Integrative Approach." In *African American Children's Mental Health: Development and Context*, edited by Nancy E. Hill, Tammy L. Mann, and Hiram E. Fitzgerald. Santa Barbara, CA: Praeger, 2011.

McCaig, Linda F., and Eric W. Nawar. "National Hospital Ambulatory Medical Survey: 2004 Emergency Department Summary." In *Advance Data from Vital and Health Statistics*. Washington, DC: Centers for Disease Control, 2006.

Miller, Joshua, and Ann Marie Garran. *Racism in the United States: Implications for the Helping Professions*. Belmont, CA: Thomson Brooks/Cole, 2008.

Miranda, J., N. Duan, C. Sherbourne, M. Schoenbaum, I. Lagomasino, M. Jackson-Triche, and K. B. Wells. "Improving Care for Minorities: Can Quality Improvement Interventions Improve Care and Outcomes for Depressed Minorities? Results of a Randomized, Controlled Trial." *Health Services Research* 38 (2003): 613–30.

Moore, Darnell. "A Pastor's Suicide: Addressing Mental Health in Black Churches." http://religiondispatches.org/a-pastors-suicide-addressing-mental-health-in-black-churches/.

Moskowitz, Gordon B., Jeff Stone, and Amanda Childs. "Implicit Stereotyping and Medical Decisions: Unconscious Stereotype Activation in Practitioners' Thoughts About African Americans." *American Journal of Public Health* 102, no. 5 (2012): 996–1001.

Mrazek, David A., John C. Hornberger, C. Anthony Altar, and Irina Degtiar. "A Review of the Clinical, Economic, and Societal Burden of Treatment-Resistant Depression: 1996–2013." *Psychiatric Services* 65, no. 8 (2014).

Murrell, Peter C. *African-Centered Pedagogy: Developing Schools of Achievement for African American Children* [in English]. Albany: State University of New York Press, 2002.

National Center for Health Statistics. "Health, United States, 2013." http://www.cdc.gov/nchs/hus/healthinsurance.htm.

———. "Health, United States, 2013: With Special Feature on Prescription Drugs." Hyattsville, MD: Centers for Disease Control and Prevention (CDC), 2014.

National Research Council and Institute of Medicine. *Preventing Mental, Emotional, and Behavioral Disorders among Young People: Progress and Possibilities.* Washington, DC: National Academies Press, 2009.

Nezu, Arthur M., Christine M. Nezu, Kelly S. Mclure, and Marni L. Zwick. "Assessment of Depression." In *Handbook of Depression*, edited by Ian H. Gotlib and Constance L. Hammen. New York: Guilford Press, 2002.

Nobles, Wade W. "African Consciousness and Liberation Struggles: Implications for the Development and Construction of Scientific Paradigms." In *Fanon Research and Development Conference*. Port of Spain, Trinidad, 1978.

———. "African Philosophy: Foundation for Black Psychology." In *Black Psychology*, edited by Reginald L. Jones. Berkeley, CA: Cobb & Henry, 1991.

NPR. *Behind Mental Health Stigmas in Black Communities.* August 20, 2012.

Oswald, Donald P., Martha J. Coutinho, Al M. Best, and Nirbhay N. Singh. "Ethnic Representation in Special Education: The Influence of School-Related Economic and Demographic Variables." *Journal of Special Education* 32, no. 4 (1999): 194–206.

Paradise, Julia, and Rachel Garfield. "What Is Medicaid's Impact on Access to Care, Health Outcomes, and Quality of Care? Setting the Record Straight on the Evidence." *Kaiser Commission on Medicaid and the Uninsured* (August 2013): 13. http://kff.org/report-section/what-is-medicaids-impact-on-access-to-care-health-outcomes-and-quality-of-care-setting-the-record-straight-on-the-evidence-issue-brief/.

Payne, January W. "Black and Blue: Depression among African-Americans." *USNews*, January 16, 2008.

Payne, Malcolm. *Modern Social Work Theory* [in English]. 4th edition. Chicago: Lyceum, 2014.

Phinney, Jean S. "When We Talk About American Ethnic Groups, What Do We Mean?" *American Psychologist* 51, no. 9 (1996): 918–27.

Poehlmann, Julie, Danielle Dallaire, Ann Booker Loper, and Leslie D. Shear. "Children's Contact with Their Incarcerated Parents: Research Findings and Recommendations." *American Psychologist* 65, no. 6 (2010): 575–98.

Primm, Annelle. "Depression and African Americans." *Journey to Wellness*, May 14, 2008.

Richardson, Elaine B. *African American Literacies* [in English]. New York: Routledge, 2003.

Roberts, A., M. S. Jackson, and I. Carlton-LaNey. "Revisiting the Need for Feminism and Afrocentric Theory When Treating African-American Female Substance Abusers." *Journal of Drug Issues* 30, no. 4 (2000): 901–17.

Roberts, Yvonne Humenay, Frank J. Snyder, Joy S. Kaufman, Meghan K. Finley, Amy Griffin, Janet Anderson, Tim Marshall, et al. "Children Exposed to the Arrest of a Family Member: Associations with Mental Health." *Journal of Child and Family Studies* 23, no. 2 (2014): 214–24.

Sherr, Michael F. "The Afrocentric Paradigm: A Pragmatic Discourse About Social Work Practice with African Americans." *Journal of Human Behavior in the Social Environment* 13, no. 3 (2006): 1–17.

Shi, Leiyu, and Douglas A. Singh. *Essentials of the U.S. Health Care System.* Burlington, MA: Jones and Bartlett, 2010.

Simms, Kevin B., Donice M. Knight, and Katherine I. Dawes. "Institutional Factors That Influence the Academic Success of African-American Men." *The Journal of Men's Studies* 1, no. 3 (1993): 253–66.

Smedley, Brian D., Adrienne Y. Stith, and Alan R. Nelson. "Unequal Treatment: Confronting Racial and Ethnic Disparities in Health Care." In *Committee on Understanding and Eliminating Racial and Ethnic Disparities in Health Care*, 29–79. Washington, DC: Institute of Medicine of the National Academies, 2002.

Snowden, Lonnie. "Barriers to Effective Mental Health Services for African Americans." *Mental Health Services Research* 3, no. 4 (2001): 181–87.

———."Bias in Mental Health Assessment and Intervention: Theory and Evidence." *American Journal of Public Health* 93, no. 2 (February 2003): 239–243.

———. "Health and Mental Health Policies' Role in Better Understanding and Closing African American–White American Disparities in Treatment Access and Quality of Care." *American Psychologist* 67, no. 7 (October 2012): 524–31.

Snowden, Lonnie R., Julia F. Hastings, and Jennifer Alvidrez. "Overrepresentation of Black Americans in Psychiatric Inpatient Care." *Psychiatric Services* 60, no. 6 (2009): 779–85.

Snowden, Lonnie R., and Ann-Marie Yamada. "Cultural Differences in Access to Care." *Annual Review of Clinical Psychology* (2005): 19–41.

Sotero, Michelle. "A Conceptual Model of Historical Trauma: Implications for Public Health Practice and Research." *Journal of Health Disparities Research and Practice* 1, no. 1 (2006): 93–108.

Sparks, Elizabeth E., and Aileen H. Parker. "The Integration of Feminism and Multiculturalism: Ethical Dilemmas at the Border." In *Practicing Feminist Ethics in Psychology*, edited by Mary M. Brabeck. Madison: University of Wisconsin Press, 2000.

Subramanyam, M. A., S. A. James, A. V. Diez-Roux, D. A. Hickson, D. Sarpong, M. Sims, H. A. Taylor Jr., and S. B. Wyatt. "Socioeconomic Status, John Henryism and Blood Pressure among African-Americans in the Jackson Heart Study." [In English]. *Social Science and Medicine* 93 (September 2013): 139–46.

Substance Abuse and Mental Health Services Administration. "Report to Congress on the Prevention and Treatment of Co-Occurring Substance Abuse Disorders and Mental Disorders." Washington, DC: U.S. Department of Health and Human Services, 2002.

Sudarkasa, Niara. "African American Families and Family Values." In *Black Families*, edited by H. P. McAdoo, 9–40. Thousand Oaks, CA: Sage Publications, 1997.

Taylor, Robert Joseph, Linda M. Chatters, Amanda Toler Woodward, and Edna Brown. "Racial and Ethnic Differences in Extended Family, Friendship, Fictive Kin, and Congregational Informal Support Networks." *Family Relations: An Interdisciplinary Journal of Applied Family Studies* 62, no. 4 (2013): 609–24.

Tucker, Catherine, and Andrea L. Dixon. "Low-Income African American Male Youth with ADHD Symptoms in the United States: Recommendations for Clinical Mental Health Counselors." *Journal of Mental Health Counseling* 31, no. 4 (2009): 309–22.

U.S. Bureau of Labor Statistics. "Unemployment Rate: Civilian Labor Force." Bureau of Labor, http://www.bls.gov/data/home.htm.

U.S. Census Bureau. "Profile American, Facts for Features—African Americans." US Census Bureau, http://www.census.gov/newsroom/releases/archives/facts_for_features_special_editions/cb13-ff02.html.

U.S. Department of Defense. "Tricare." http://www.tricare.mil.

U.S. Department of Health and Human Services. "Mental Health: A Report of the Surgeon General." Rockville, MD: U.S. Department of Health and Human Services, Substance Abuse and Mental Health Services Administration, Center for Mental Health Services, National Institutes of Health, National Institute of Mental Health, 1999.

———. "Mental Health: Culture, Race, and Ethnicity—A Supplement to Mental Health: A Report of the Surgeon General." Rockville, MD: U.S. Department of Health and Human Services, Public Health Service, Office of the Surgeon General, 2001.

Vaz, Kim Marie. "Reflecting Team Group Therapy and Its Congruence with Feminist Principles: A Focus on African American Women." *Women & Therapy* 28, no. 2 (2005): 65–75.

Whipple, Sara Sepanski, Gary W. Evans, Rachel L. Barry, and Lorraine E. Maxwell. "An Ecological Perspective on Cumulative School and Neighborhood Risk Factors Related to Achievement." *Journal of Applied Developmental Psychology* 31, no. 6 (2010): 422–27.

Williams, Carmen Braun. "Counseling African American Women: Multiple Identities—Multiple Constraints." *Journal of Counseling & Development* 83, no. 3 (2005): 278–83.

Williams, David R., and Chiquita Collins. "Racial Residential Segregation: A Fundamental Cause of Racial Disparities in Health." *Public Health Reports* 116, no. 5 (2001): 404–16.

Williams, David R., Hector M. Gonzalez, Harold W. Neighbors, Randy Nesse, Jamie M. Abelson, Julie Sweetman, and James S. Jackson. "Prevalence and Distribution of Major Depressive Disorder in African Americans, Caribbean Blacks, and Non-Hispanic Whites: Results from the National Survey of American Life (NSAL)." *Archives of General Psychiatry* 64 (2007): 305–15.

Williams, David R., and S. A. Mohammed. "Racism and Health I: Pathways and Scientific Evidence." [In English]. *American Behavioral Scientist* 57, no. 8 (2013): 1152–73.

Williams, David R., Harold W. Neighbors, and James S. Jackson. "Racial/Ethnic Discrimination and Health: Findings from Community Studies." *American Journal of Public Health* 93, no. 2 (2003): 200–8.

Williams, David R., and Ruth Williams-Morris. "Racism and Mental Health: The African American Experience." *Ethnicity & Health* 5, no. 3/4 (2000): 243–68.

Williams, J. W., Jr., C. A. Kerber, C. D. Mulrow, A. Medina, and C. Aguilar. "Depressive Disorders in Primary Care: Prevalence, Functional Disability, and Identification." *Journal of General Internal Medicine* 10, no. 1 (1995): 7–12.

Williams, Terrie M. *Black Pain: It Just Looks Like We're Not Hurting: Real Talk for When There's Nowhere to Go but Up* [in English]. New York: Scribner, 2008.

———. *Black Pain: It Just Looks Like We're Not Hurting*. New York: Scribner, 2009.

Wilson, William Julius. *More Than Just Race: Being Black and Poor in the Inner City (Issues of Our Time)*. New York: W. W. Norton & Company, 2010.

Wood, Dana, Rachel Kaplan, and Vonnie C. McLoyd. "Gender Differences in the Educational Expectations of Urban, Low-Income African American Youth: The Role of Parents and the School." *Journal of Youth and Adolescence* 36, no. 4 (2007): 417–27.

Yeager, Kenneth, David Cutler, Dale Svendsen, and Grayce M. Sills, eds. *Modern Community Mental Health: An Interdisciplinary Approach*. New York: Oxford University Press, 2013.

Yu, Yan, and David R. Williams. "Socioeconomic Status and Mental Health." In *Handbook of the Sociology of Mental Health*, edited by Carol S. Aneshensel and Jo C. Phelan, 151–66. New York: Kluwer Academic, 1999.

Zlotnick, Caron, Sheri L. Johnson, Ivan W. Miller, Teri Pearlstein, and Margaret Howard. "Postpartum Depression in Women Receiving Public Assistance: Pilot Study of an Interpersonal-Therapy-Oriented Group Intervention." *American Journal of Psychiatry* 158, no. 4 (2001): 638–40.

Zlotnick, Caron, Ivan Miller, Teri Pearlstein, Margaret Howard, and Patrick Sweeney. "A Preventive Intervention for Pregnant Women on Public Assistance at Risk for Postpartum Depression." *American Journal of Psychiatry* 163, no. 8 (2006): 1443–45.

Notes

PREFACE

1. Centers for Disease Control and Prevention, "Minority Health: Black or African American Populations," http://www.cdc.gov/minorityhealth/populations/remp/black.html.

2. James S. Jackson, Cleopatra Howard Caldwell, and Sherrill L. Sellers, eds., *Researching Black Communities: A Methodological Guide* (Ann Arbor, MI: University of Michigan Press, 2012).

1. UNDERSTANDING THE SIGNS OF DEPRESSION

1. U.S. Census Bureau, "Profile American, Facts for Features—African Americans," http://www.census.gov/newsroom/facts-for-features/2015/cb15-ff01.html.

2. Carmen DeNavas-Walt, Bernadette D. Proctor, and Jessica C. Smith, *Income, Poverty, and Health Insurance Coverage in the United States: 2012*, ed. U.S. Census Bureau (Washington, DC: U.S. Government Printing Office, 2013).

3. James S. Jackson, Cleopatra Howard Caldwell, and Sherrill L. Sellers, eds., *Researching Black Communities: A Methodological Guide* (Ann Arbor, MI: University of Michigan Press, 2012).

4. M. A. Subramanyam et al., "Socioeconomic Status, John Henryism and Blood Pressure among African-Americans in the Jackson Heart Study," *Social Science and Medicine* 93 (2013): 139–46.

5. Sherman A. James, "John Henryism and the Health of African Americans," *Culture, Medicine and Psychiatry* 18 (1994): 163–82.

6. Yan Yu and David R. Williams, "Socioeconomic Status and Mental Health," in *Handbook of the Sociology of Mental Health*, ed. Carol S. Aneshensel and Jo C. Phelan (New York: Kluwer Academic, 1999).

7. D. R. Williams and S. A. Mohammed, "Racism and Health I: Pathways and Scientific Evidence," *American Behavioral Scientist* 57, no. 8 (2013).

8. H. M. Gonzalez et al., "Depression Care in the United States: Too Little for Too Few," *Archives of General Psychiatry* 67, no. 1 (2010): 37–46.

9. S. Assari, "Chronic Medical Conditions and Major Depressive Disorder: Differential Role of Positive Religious Coping among African Americans, Caribbean Blacks and Non-Hispanic Whites," *International Journal of Preventive Medicine* 5, no. 4 (2014): 405–13.

10. Terrie M. Williams, *Black Pain: It Just Looks Like We're Not Hurting* (New York: Scribner, 2009).

11. A. A. Agyemang et al., "Quality of Depression Treatment in Black Americans with Major Depression and Comorbid Medical Illness," *General Hospital Psychiatry* 36, no. 4 (2014): 431–36.

12. Ian H. Gotlib and Constance L. Hammen, eds., *Handbook of Depression*, third ed. (New York: Guilford Press, 2014).

13. American Psychiatric Association, ed., *Diagnostic and Statistical Manual of Mental Disorders (DSM-V)*, fifth ed. (Arlington, VA: American Psychiatric Publishing, 2013).

14. Julia F. Hastings, "Understanding Diabetes and Depression among African Americans in California and New York" (California and New York: National Institute on Minority Health and Health Disparities [NIMHD], 2014).

15. David R. Williams et al., "Prevalence and Distribution of Major Depressive Disorder in African Americans, Caribbean Blacks, and Non-Hispanic Whites: Results from the National Survey of American Life (NSAL)," *Archives of General Psychiatry* 64 (2007).

16. James S. Jackson et al., "The National Survey of American Life: A Study of Racial, Ethnic, and Cultural Influences on Mental Disorders and Mental Health," *International Journal of Methods in Psychiatric Research* 13, no. 4 (2004): 196–207.

17. Williams et al., "Prevalence and Distribution of Major Depressive Disorder in African Americans, Caribbean Blacks, and Non-Hispanic Whites."

18. U.S. Department of Health and Human Services, Centers for Disease Control and Prevention, National Center for Health Statistics, "Health, United States, 2013: With Special Feature on Prescription Drugs" (Hyattsville, MD: Centers for Disease Control [CDC], 2014).

19. Institute of Medicine, *Unequal Treatment: Confronting Racial and Ethnic Disparities in Health Care*, ed. Institute of Medicine and Brian D. Smedley, Adrienne Y. Stith, and Alan R. Nelson (Washington, DC: The National Academies Press, 2002).

20. Gotlib and Hammen, *Handbook of Depression*.

21. Gotlib and Hammen, *Handbook of Depression*.

22. Assari, "Chronic Medical Conditions and Major Depressive Disorder."

23. John Head, *Black Men and Depression: Saving Our Lives, Healing Our Families and Friends* (New York: Crown Publishing Group, 2010).

24. Head, *Black Men and Depression*.

25. Gotlib and Hammen, *Handbook of Depression*.

26. Gotlib and Hammen, *Handbook of Depression*.

27. U.S. Department of Health and Human Services, "Mental Health: Culture, Race, and Ethnicity—a Supplement to Mental Health: A Report of the Surgeon General" (Rockville, MD: U.S. Department of Health and Human Services, Public Health Service, Office of the Surgeon General, 2001).

28. Brian D. Smedley, Adrienne Y. Stith, and Alan R. Nelson, "Unequal Treatment: Confronting Racial and Ethnic Disparities in Health Care," in *Unequal Treatment: Confronting Racial and Ethnic Disparities in Health Care* (Washington, DC: Institute of Medicine of the National Academies, 2003).

29. Joshua Breslau et al., "Lifetime Risk and Persistence of Psychiatric Disorders across Ethnic Groups in the United States," *Psychological Medicine* 35, no. 3 (2005): 317–27.

30. U.S. Department of Health and Human Services, "Mental Health: Culture, Race, and Ethnicity."

31. U.S. Department of Health and Human Services, "Mental Health: Culture, Race, and Ethnicity."

32. Lonnie R. Snowden and Ann-Marie Yamada, "Cultural Differences in Access to Care," *Annual Review of Clinical Psychology* (2005): 143–66.

33. Paul E. Greenberg et al., "The Economic Burden of Depression in the United States: How Did It Change between 1990 and 2000?" *Journal of Clinical Psychiatry* 64, no. 12 (2003): 1465–75.

34. David A. Mrazek et al., "A Review of the Clinical, Economic, and Societal Burden of Treatment-Resistant Depression: 1996–2013," *Psychiatric Services* 65, no. 8 (2014): 977–87.

35. D. M. Herbeck et al., "Variations in Use of Second Generation Antipsychotic Medication by Race among Adult Psychiatric Patients," *Psychiatric Services* 55, no. 6 (2004): 677–84.

36. U.S. Department of Health and Human Services, "Mental Health: Culture, Race, and Ethnicity."

37. L. R. Snowden, "Health and Mental Health Policies' Role in Better Understanding and Closing African American-White American Disparities in Treatment Access and Quality of Care," *American Psychologist* 67, no. 7 (2012): 524–31.

38. William Julius Wilson, *More Than Just Race: Being Black and Poor in the Inner City (Issues of Our Time)* (New York: W. W. Norton & Company, 2010).

39. Wilson, *More Than Just Race.*

40. Martha J. Bailey and Sheldon Danziger, eds., *Legacies of the War on Poverty*, The National Poverty Center Series on Poverty and Public Policy (New York: Russell Sage Foundation, 2013).

41. Institute of Medicine, "Emergency Medical Services at the Crossroads" (Washington, DC, 2006).

42. Linda F. McCaig and Eric W. Nawar, "National Hospital Ambulatory Medical Survey: 2004 Emergency Department Summary," in *Advance Data from Vital and Health Statistics* (Centers for Disease Control, 2006).

43. U.S. Department of Health and Human Services, "Mental Health: A Report of the Surgeon General" (Rockville, MD: U.S. Department of Health and Human Services, Substance Abuse and Mental Health Services Administration, Center for Mental Health Services, National Institutes of Health, National Institute of Mental Health, 1999).

44. Seth Kunen et al., "Race Disparities in Psychiatric Rates in Emergency Departments," *Journal of Consulting and Clinical Psychology* 73, no. 1 (2005): 116–26.

45. Kenneth P. Lindsey and Gordon L. Paul, "Involuntary Commitments to Public Mental Illness Issues Involving the Overrepresentation of Blacks and Assessment of Relevant Functioning," *Psychological Bulletin* 106, no. 2 (1989): 171–83.

46. Lonnie R. Snowden, Julia F. Hastings, and Jennifer Alvidrez, "Overrepresentation of Black Americans in Psychiatric Inpatient Care," *Psychiatric Services* 60, no. 6 (2009): 779–85; D. M. Griffith et al., "Ethnicity, Nativity, and the Health of American Blacks," *Journal of Health Care for the Poor and Underserved* 22, no. 1 (2011); L. A. Martin, H. W. Neighbors, and D. M. Griffith, "The Experience of Symptoms of Depression in Men vs. Women: Analysis of the National Comorbidity Survey Replication," *JAMA Psychiatry* 70, no. 10 (2013); D. L. Hudson et al., "The Relationship between Socioeconomic Position and Depression among a US Nationally Representative Sample of African Americans," *Social Psychiatry in Epidemiology* 47, no. 3 (2012): 373–81.

2. PERMISSION TO HEAL

1. Center for Behavioral Health Statistics and Quality, "Results from the 2012 National Survey on Drug Use and Health: Summary of National Findings" (Rockville, MD: Substance Abuse and Mental Health Services Administration, 2013).

2. NPR, *Behind Mental Health Stigmas in Black Communities*, August 20, 2012.

3. Lani V. Jones et al., "A Qualitative Study of Black Women's Experiences in Drug Abuse and Mental Health Services," *Affilia* (2014).

4. bell hooks, *Sisters of the Yam: Black Women and Self-Recovery* (Cambridge, MA: South End Press, 2005).

5. Arthur M. Nezu, Christine M. Nezu, Kelly S. Mclure, and Marni L. Zwick, "Assessment of Depression," in *Handbook of Depression*, ed. Ian H. Gotlib and Constance L. Hammen (New York: Guilford Press, 2002).

6. Nezu et al., "Assessment of Depression."

7. Jones et al., "A Qualitative Study of Black Women's Experiences"; Nancy Boyd-Franklin et al., *Therapy in the Real World: Effective Treatments for Challenging Problems* (New York: Guilford Press, 2013).

8. Jones et al., "A Qualitative Study of Black Women's Experiences"; Boyd Franklin et al., *Therapy in the Real World*; David R. Williams, Harold W. Neighbors, and James S. Jackson, "Racial/Ethnic Discrimination and Health: Findings from Community Studies," *American Journal of Public Health* 93, no. 2 (2003).

9. J. W. Williams Jr. et al., "Depressive Disorders in Primary Care: Prevalence, Functional Disability, and Identification," *Journal of General Internal Medicine* 10, no. 1 (1995).

10. Jones et al., "A Qualitative Study of Black Women's Experiences."

11. Jones et al., "A Qualitative Study of Black Women's Experiences"; Michelle Sotero, "A Conceptual Model of Historical Trauma: Implications for Public Health Practice and Research," *Journal of Health Disparities Research and Practice* 1, no. 1 (2006); Nancy Boyd-Franklin, "Recurrent Themes in the Treatment of African American Women in Group Therapy," *Women & Therapy* 11 (2003).

12. John Head, *Black Men and Depression: Understanding and Overcoming Depression in Black Men* (New York: Harlem Moon/Broadway Books, 2005).

13. Boyd-Franklin, "Recurrent Themes in the Treatment of African American Women in Group Therapy."

14. Boyd-Franklin, "Recurrent Themes in the Treatment of African American Women in Group Therapy"; January W. Payne, "Black and Blue: Depression among African-Americans," *USNews*, January 16, 2008.

15. Toni Cade Bambara, *The Salt Eaters* (New York: Random House, 1980).

16. Boyd-Franklin et al., *Therapy in the Real World*.

17. Nezu et al., "Assessment of Depression"; Substance Abuse and Mental Health Services Administration, "Report to Congress on the Prevention and Treatment of Co-Occurring Substance Abuse Disorders and Mental Disorders" (U.S. Department of Health and Human Services, 2002); Terrie M. Williams, *Black Pain: It Just Looks Like We're Not Hurting: Real Talk for When There's Nowhere to Go But Up* (New York: Scribner, 2008).

18. Williams, *Black Pain*; U.S. Department of Health and Human Services, "Mental Health: Culture, Race, and Ethnicity—a Supplement to Mental Health: A Report of the Surgeon General" (Rockville, MD: U.S. Department of Health and Human Services, Mental Health Services Administration, Center for Mental Health Services, 2001); June G. Hopps and Elaine Pinderhughes, *Group Work with Overwhelmed Clients: How the Power of Groups Can Help People Transform Their Lives* (New York: Free Press, 1999).

19. David R. Williams, Harold W. Neighbors, and James S. Jackson, "Racial/Ethnic Discrimination and Health: Findings from Community Studies," *American Journal of Public Health* 93, no. 2 (2003); U.S. Department of Health and Human Services, "Mental Health"; Lonnie Snowden, "Barriers to Effective Mental Health Services for African Americans," *Mental Health Services Research* 3, no. 4 (2001).

20. Snowden, "Barriers to Effective Mental Health Services for African Americans."

21. The Carter Center, "The President's New Freedom Commission on Mental Health: Transforming the Vision," in *The Nineteenth Annual Rosalynn Carter Symposium on Mental Health Policy* (2003).

22. Snowden, "Barriers to Effective Mental Health Services for African Americans"; S. L. Bowie and D. M. Dopwell, "Metastressors as Barriers to Self-Sufficiency among TANF-Reliant African American and Latina Women," *Affilia: Journal of Women and Social Work* 28, no. 2 (2013); N. G. Choi and J. M. Gonzalez, "Geriatric Mental Health Clinicians' Perceptions of Barriers and Contributors to Retention of Older Minorities in Treatment: An Exploratory Study," *Clinical Gerontologist* 28, no. 3 (2005).

23. Jones et al., "A Qualitative Study of Black Women's Experiences in Drug Abuse and Mental Health Services"; Nia Hamm, "Black Folks and Mental Health: Why Do We Suffer in Silence?" *Ebony*, October 1, 2012; Joyce A. Ladner, "Introduction to Tomorrow's Tomorrow: The Black Woman," in *Feminism & Methodology*, ed. Sandra Harding (Bloomington, IN: Indiana University Press, 1987).

24. Jones et al., "A Qualitative Study of Black Women's Experiences in Drug Abuse and Mental Health Services"; Ladner, "Introduction to Tomorrow's Tomorrow."

25. Jones et al., "A Qualitative Study of Black Women's Experiences in Drug Abuse and Mental Health Services."

26. Bambara, *The Salt Eaters*.

27. Annelle Primm, "Depression and African Americans," *Journey to Wellness*, May 14, 2008.

28. Eleanor H. Hoytt and Hilary Beard, *Health First! The Black Woman's Wellness Guide* (New York: Smiley Books, 2012).

29. Williams Jr. et al., "Depressive Disorders in Primary Care."

30. Nezu et al., "Assessment of Depression."

31. Hopps and Pinderhughes, *Group Work with Overwhelmed Clients*; Lorraine M. Gutierrez, "Working with Women of Color: An Empowerment Perspective," *Social Work* 35, no. 2 (1990); Kim Marie Vaz, "Reflecting Team Group Therapy and Its Congruence with Feminist Principles: A Focus on African American Women," *Women & Therapy* 28, no. 2 (2005).

32. Nezu et al., "Assessment of Depression."

33. Jones et al., "A Qualitative Study of Black Women's Experiences in Drug Abuse and Mental Health Services."

34. Nezu et al., "Assessment of Depression."

35. Nezu et al., "Assessment of Depression."

36. Malcolm Payne, *Modern Social Work Theory*, 4th ed. (Chicago: Lyceum, 2014).

37. Gutierrez, "Working with Women of Color."

38. Boyd-Franklin et al., *Therapy in the Real World*; Gutierrez, "Working with Women of Color."

39. Nezu et al., "Assessment of Depression"; Gutierrez, "Working with Women of Color"; Therese J. Borchard, "6 Steps for Beating Depression," http://psychcentral.com/blog/archives/2009/07/09/6-steps-for-beating-depression/; Hamm, "Black Folks and Mental Health."

40. Gutierrez, "Working with Women of Color."

41. Charles Husband, "Recognising Diversity and Developing Skills: The Proper Role of Transcultural Communication," *European Journal of Social Work* 3, no. 3 (2000).

42. Jones et al., "A Qualitative Study of Black Women's Experiences in Drug Abuse and Mental Health Services"; Sotero, "A Conceptual Model of Historical Trauma"; Boyd-Franklin, "Recurrent Themes in the Treatment of African American Women in Group Therapy"; Payne, *Modern Social Work Theory*.

43. Na'im Akbar, "The Evolution of Human Psychology for African Americans," in *Black Psychology*, ed. Reginald L. Jones (Berkeley, CA: Cobb & Henry, 1991).

44. Na'im Akbar, "Africentric Social Sciences for Human Liberation," *Journal of Black Studies* 14, no. 4 (1984); Wade W. Nobles, "African Consciousness and Liberation Struggles: Implications for the Development and Construction of Scientific Paradigms," in *Fanon Research and Development Conference* (Port of Spain, Trinidad, 1978); Jacob Carruthers, "Towards the Development of a Black Social Theory," in *Howard University Graduate Student Council's Distinguished Lecture Series* (Washington, DC, 1989).

45. Husband, "Recognising Diversity and Developing Skills"; Akbar, "The Evolution of Human Psychology for African Americans"; Akbar, "Africentric Social Sciences for Human Liberation"; D. J. Gilbert, A. R. Harvey, and F. Z. Belgrave, "Advancing the Africentric Paradigm Shift Discourse: Building toward Evidence-Based Africentric Interventions in Social Work Practice with African Americans," *Social Work* 54, no. 3 (2009).

46. Borchard, "6 Steps for Beating Depression"; Aminifu R. Harvey and Robert B. Hill, "Africentric Youth and Family Rites of Passage Program: Promoting Resilience among at-Risk African American Youths," *Social Work* 49, no. 1 (2004); Michael F. Sherr, "The Afrocentric Paradigm: A Pragmatic Discourse About Social Work Practice with African Americans," *Journal of Human Behavior in the Social Environment* 13, no. 3 (2006); Wade W. Nobles, "African Philosophy: Foundation for Black Psychology," in *Black Psychology*, ed. Reginald L. Jones (Berkeley, CA: Cobb & Henry, 1991).

47. Jones et al., "A Qualitative Study of Black Women's Experiences in Drug Abuse and Mental Health Services."

48. Phillippe B. Cunningham, Sharon L. Foster, and Sarah E. Warner, "Culturally Relevant Family-Based Treatment for Adolescent Delinquency and Substance Abuse: Understanding Within-Session Processes," *Journal of Clinical Psychology* 66, no. 8 (2010).
49. Janet E. Helms, "An Update of Helms's White and People of Color Racial Identity Models," in *Handbook of Multicultural Counseling*, ed. Joseph G. Ponterotto et al. (Thousand Oaks, CA: Sage Publications, 1995); Jean S. Phinney, "When We Talk About American Ethnic Groups, What Do We Mean?" *American Psychologist* 51, no. 9 (1996).
50. Elizabeth E. Sparks and Aileen H. Parker, "The Integration of Feminism and Multiculturalism: Ethical Dilemmas at the Border," in *Practicing Feminist Ethics in Psychology*, ed. Mary M. Brabeck (Madison: University of Wisconsin Press, 2000); Lani V. Jones and Briggett Ford, "Depression in African American Women: Application of a Psychosocial Competence Practice Framework," *Affilia* 23, no. 2 (2008).
51. Nancy Boyd-Franklin, "Incorporating Spirituality and Religion into the Treatment of African American Clients," *Counseling Psychologist* 38, no. 7 (2010); Beverly Greene, "Psychotherapy with African American Women: Integrating Feminist and Psychodynamic Models," *Smith College Studies in Social Work* 67, no. 3 (1997).
52. Boyd-Franklin, "Recurrent Themes in the Treatment of African American Women in Group Therapy"; A. Roberts, M. S. Jackson, and I. Carlton-LaNey, "Revisiting the Need for Feminism and Afrocentric Theory When Treating African-American Female Substance Abusers," *Journal of Drug Issues* 30, no. 4 (2000); Carmen Braun Williams, "Counseling African American Women: Multiple Identities—Multiple Constraints," *Journal of Counseling & Development* 83, no. 3 (2005).
53. Leslie C. Jackson, and Beverly Greene, "Review of Psychotherapy with African American Women: Innovations in Psychodynamic Perspectives and Practices," *The Psychoanaylitic Quarterly* 72 (2003).
54. Joshua Miller, and Ann Marie Garran. *Racism in the United States: Implications for the Helping Professions*. Belmont, CA: Thomson Brooks/Cole, 2008.
55. Lonnie R. Snowden, "Bias in Mental Health Assessment and Intervention: Theory and Evidence," *American Journal of Public Health* 93, no. 2 (February 2003): 239-243.
56. Lani V. Jones, and Briggett Ford, "Depression in African American Women."
57. Bambara, *The Salt Eaters*.

3. DEALING WITH MENTAL ILLNESS

1. Kenneth Yeager et al., eds., *Modern Community Mental Health: An Interdisciplinary Approach* (New York: Oxford University Press, 2013).
2. Yeager, *Modern Community Mental Health*.
3. American Psychological Association, *APA Dictionary of Psychology* (Washington, DC: American Psychological Association, 2007).
4. National Alliance on Mental Illness, accessed July 1, 2014, http://www.nami.org/.
5. National Alliance on Mental Illness.
6. Community Tool Box, http://ctb.ku.edu/en.
7. Niara Sudarkasa, "African American Families and Family Values," in *Black Families* (Thousand Oaks, CA: Sage Publications, 1997).
8. Kenneth Heller, Richard J. Viken, and Ralph W. Swindle, "What Do Network Members Know? Network Members as Reporters of Depression among Caucasian-American and African-American Older Women," *Aging & Mental Health* 17, no. 2 (2013): 215–25.
9. Heller et al., "What Do Network Members Know?"
10. David R. Williams, Hector González, Harold Neighbors, Randolph Nesse, Jamie M. Abelson, Julie Sweetman, and James S. Jackson, "Prevalence and Distribution of Major Depressive Disorder in African Americans, Caribbean Blacks, and Non-Hispanic Whites: Results from the National Survey of American Life," *Archives of General Psychiatry* 64, no. 3 (2007): 305–15.

11. Agnes Martin, Noreen Boadi, Caroline Fernandes, Sherry Watt, and Tracy Robinson-Wood, "Applying Resistance Theory to Depression in Black Women," *Journal of Systemic Therapies* 32, no. 1 (2013): 1–13.

12. Marjorie Beeghly et al., "Prevalence, Stability, and Socio-Demographic Correlates of Depressive Symptoms in Black Mothers during the First 18 Months Postpartum," *Maternal and Child Health Journal* 7, no. 3 (2003).

13. Beeghly et al., "Prevalence, Stability, and Socio-Demographic Correlates."

14. Robert Joseph Taylor et al., "Racial and Ethnic Differences in Extended Family, Friendship, Fictive Kin, and Congregational Informal Support Networks," *Family Relations: An Interdisciplinary Journal of Applied Family Studies* 62, no. 4 (2013).

15. C. Eric Lincoln and Lawrence H. Mamiya, *The Black Church in the African-American Experience* (Durham: Duke University Press, 1990).

16. Daphne C. Watkins, B. Lee Green, Brian M. Rivers, and Kyrel L. Rowell, "Depression and Black Men: Implications for Future Research," *Journal of Men's Health & Gender* 3, no. 3 (2006): 227–35.

17. Wizdom Powell Hammond, "Taking It Like a Man: Masculine Role Norms as Moderators of the Racial Discrimination-Depressive Symptoms Association among African American Men," *American Journal of Public Health* 102, no. S2 (2012): S232–S241.

18. Sean Joe, "Implications of Focusing on Black Youth Self-Destructive Behaviors Instead of Suicide When Designing Preventative Interventions," in *Reducing Adolescent Risk: Toward an Integrated Approach*, ed. Daniel Romer (Thousand Oaks, CA: Sage Publications, 2003).

19. Charis E. Kubrin and Tim Wadsworth, "Explaining Suicide among Blacks and Whites: How Socioeconomic Factors and Gun Availability Affect Race-Specific Suicide Rates," *Social Science Quarterly* 90, no. 5 (2009).

20. Sean Joe and Mark S. Kaplan, "Firearm-Related Suicide among Young African-American Males," *Psychiatric Services* 53, no. 3 (2002).

21. Sean Joe, "Implications of National Suicide Trends for Social Work Practice with Black Youth," *Child and Adolescent Social Work Journal* 23, no. 4 (2006).

22. Harvard School of Public Health, "Guns & Suicide: The Hidden Toll," accessed September 27, 2014, http://www.hsph.harvard.edu/magazine-features/guns-and-suicide-the-hidden-toll/.

23. Robert Davis, "Suicide among Young Blacks: Trends and Perspectives," *Phylon (1960)* 41, no. 3 (1980).

24. Sean Joe, "Suicide among African Americans: A Male's Burden," in *Social Work with African American Males: Health, Mental Health, and Social Policy*, ed. Waldo E. Johnson (New York: Oxford University Press, 2010).

25. Lincoln and Mamiya, *The Black Church in the African American Experience.*

26. Andrew Billingsley, *Mighty Like a River: The Black Church and Social Reform* (New York: Oxford University Press, 1999).

27. Darnell Moore, "A Pastor's Suicide: Addressing Mental Health in Black Churches," http://religiondispatches.org/a-pastors-suicide-addressing-mental-health-in-black-churches/.

28. Lincoln and Mamiya, *The Black Church in the African American Experience.*

29. Dale P. Andrews, *Practical Theology for Black Churches: Bridging Black Theology and African American Folk Religion* (Louisville, KY: Westminster John Knox Press, 2002).

30. Pamela Martin, "Theology and Faith Development among African American Adolescents: An Integrative Approach," in *African American Children's Mental Health: Development and Context*, ed. Nancy E. Hill, Tammy L. Mann, and Hiram E. Fitzgerald (Santa Barbara, CA: Praeger, 2011).

31. Yvonne Humenay Roberts et al., "Children Exposed to the Arrest of a Family Member: Associations with Mental Health," *Journal of Child and Family Studies* 23, no. 2 (2014).

32. David J. Kolko et al., "Posttraumatic Stress Symptoms in Children and Adolescents Referred for Child Welfare Investigation: A National Sample of In-Home and Out-of-Home Care," *Child Maltreatment* 15, no. 1 (2010).

33. Julie Poehlmann et al., "Children's Contact with Their Incarcerated Parents: Research Findings and Recommendations," *American Psychologist* 65, no. 6 (2010).

34. Marc S. Atkins et al., "Toward the Integration of Education and Mental Health in Schools," *Administration and Policy in Mental Health and Mental Health Services Research* 37, no. 1–2 (2010).

35. Sara Sepanski Whipple et al., "An Ecological Perspective on Cumulative School and Neighborhood Risk Factors Related to Achievement," *Journal of Applied Developmental Psychology* 31, no. 6 (2010).

36. John L. Hosp and Daniel J. Reschly, "Disproportionate Representation of Minority Students in Special Education: Academic, Demographic, and Economic Predictors," *Exceptional Children* 70, no. 2 (2004).

37. Jo M. Hendrickson et al., "Decision Making Factors Associated with Placement of Students with Emotional and Behavioral Disorders in Restrictive Educational Settings," *Education and Treatment of Children* 21, no. 3 (1998).

38. Donald P. Oswald et al., "Ethnic Representation in Special Education: The Influence of School-Related Economic and Demographic Variables," *The Journal of Special Education* 32, no. 4 (1999).

39. Revathy Arunkumar, Carol Midgley, and Tim Urdan, "Perceiving High or Low Home-School Dissonance: Longitudinal Effects on Adolescent Emotional and Academic Well-Being," *Journal of Research on Adolescence* 9, no. 4 (1999).

40. Judith S. Brook et al., "Personality, Family, and Ecological Influences on Adolescent Drug Use: A Developmental Analysis," *Journal of Chemical Dependency Treatment* 1, no. 2 (1988).

41. A. Wade Boykin and Forrest D. Toms, "Black Child Socialization: A Conceptual Framework," in *Black Children: Social, Educational, and Parental Environments*, ed. Harriette Pipes McAdoo and John Lewis McAdoo (Beverly Hills: Sage Publications, 1985).

42. Carol D. Lee, "Is October Brown Chinese? A Cultural Modeling Activity System for Underachieving Students," *American Educational Research Journal* 38, no. 1 (2001).

43. "Cultural Modeling: Chat as a Lens for Understanding Instructional Discourse Based on African American English Discourse Patterns," in *Vygotsky's Educational Theory in Cultural Context*, ed. Alex Kozulin (New York: Cambridge University Press, 2003).

44. Peter C. Murrell, *African-Centered Pedagogy: Developing Schools of Achievement for African American Children* (Albany: State University of New York Press, 2002).

45. Elaine B. Richardson, *African American Literacies* (New York: Routledge, 2003).

46. Marvin Lynn, "Race, Culture, and the Education of African Americans," *Educational Theory* 56, no. 1 (2006).

47. Kubrin and Wadsworth, "Explaining Suicide among Blacks and Whites: How Socioeconomic Factors and Gun Availability Affect Race-Specific Suicide Rates."

48. Catherine Tucker and Andrea L. Dixon, "Low-Income African American Male Youth with ADHD Symptoms in the United States: Recommendations for Clinical Mental Health Counselors," *Journal of Mental Health Counseling* 31, no. 4 (2009).

49. David R. Williams and Chiquita Collins, "Racial Residential Segregation: A Fundamental Cause of Racial Disparities in Health," *Public Health Reports* 116, no. 5 (2001).

50. David R. Williams and Ruth Williams-Morris, "Racism and Mental Health: The African American Experience," *Ethnicity & Health* 5, no. 3/4 (2000).

51. Jan Hughes and Oi-man Kwok, "Influence of Student-Teacher and Parent-Teacher Relationships on Lower Achieving Readers' Engagement and Achievement in the Primary Grades," *Journal of Educational Psychology* 99, no. 1 (2007).

52. Dana Wood, Rachel Kaplan, and Vonnie C. McLoyd, "Gender Differences in the Educational Expectations of Urban, Low-Income African American Youth: The Role of Parents and the School," *Journal of Youth and Adolescence* 36, no. 4 (2007).

53. Antoine M. Garibaldi, "Educating and Motivating African American Males to Succeed," *The Journal of Negro Education* 61, no. 1 (1992).

54. Kevin B. Simms, Donice M. Knight, and Katherine I. Dawes, "Institutional Factors That Influence the Academic Success of African-American Men," *Journal of Men's Studies* 1, no. 3 (1993).

55. Wood, "Gender Differences in the Educational Expectations of Urban, Low-Income African American Youth."

56. Centers for Disease Control and Prevention, "Depression in the U.S. Household Population, 2009–2012," http://www.cdc.gov/nchs/pressroom/upcoming.htm.

57. Kaiser Commission on Medicaid and the Uninsured, "Fact Sheet Health Coverage by Race and Ethnicity: The Potential Impact of the Affordable Care Act Executive Summary," http://kaiserfamilyfoundation.files.wordpress.com/2014/07/8423-health-coverage-by-race-and-ethnicity.pdf.

58. Carla Boutin-Foster et al., "Ethical Considerations for Conducting Health Disparities Research in Community Health Centers: A Social-Ecological Perspective," *American Journal of Public Health* 103, no. 12 (2013).

59. Urie Bronfenbrenner, "Contexts of Child Rearing: Problems and Prospects," *American Psychologist* 34, no. 10 (1979).

60. Urie Bronfenbrenner, *Making Human Beings Human: Bioecological Perspectives on Human Development* (Newbury Park, CA: Sage, 2005).

61. Bronfenbrenner, "Contexts of Child Rearing."

62. Bronfenbrenner, *Making Human Beings Human.*

63. Gordon B. Moskowitz, Jeff Stone, and Amanda Childs, "Implicit Stereotyping and Medical Decisions: Unconscious Stereotype Activation in Practitioners' Thoughts About African Americans," *American Journal of Public Health* 102, no. 5 (2012).

64. Bronfenbrenner, "Contexts of Child Rearing."

65. Bronfenbrenner, *Making Human Beings Human.*

66. National Alliance on Mental Illness, accessed July 1, 2014,http://www.nami.org/.

67. Mental Health Ministries, accessed September 27, 2014, http://www.mentalhealthministries.net/.

68. Adelle M. Banks, "No Longer behind the Curve: Black Churches Address Mental Illness, accessed September 27, 2014, http://www.religionnews.com/2014/08/14/longer-behind-curve-black-churches-address-mental-illness/.

69. Memphis Healing Center, accessed September 27, 2014, http://www.memphishealingcenter.com/emotional.html.

70. NYU Langone School of Medicine Center for Early Childhood Health and Development (CEHD)—Health and Behavior, accessed October 2, 2014, http://pophealth.med.nyu.edu/divisions/cehd/parentcorps.

71. NYU Langone School of Medicine Center for Early Childhood Health and Development (CEHD).

72. NYU Langone School of Medicine Media Relations, accessed October 2, 2014, http://communications.med.nyu.edu/media-relations/news/parentcorps-helps-children-do-better-school.

73. NYU Langone School of Medicine Media Relations.

74. Centers for Disease Control and Prevention, accessed September 27, 2014, http://www.cdc.gov/prc/pdf/boys-health-risks-reduced-father-son-bonds.pdf.

75. Eric Schulzke, "Too Few Men Leads to Youth Violence, University of Michigan Study Finds," *Deseret News National*, accessed September 27, 2014, http://national.deseretnews.com/article/793/Too-few-men-leads-to-youth-violence-University-of-Michigan-study-finds.html.

76. Caron Zlotnick et al., "Postpartum Depression in Women Receiving Public Assistance: Pilot Study of an Interpersonal-Therapy-Oriented Group Intervention," *American Journal of Psychiatry* 158, no. 4 (2001).

77. Caron Zlotnick et al., "A Preventive Intervention for Pregnant Women on Public Assistance at Risk for Postpartum Depression," *Journal of Psychiatry* 163, no. 8 (2006).

78. Kathy Crockett et al., "A Depression Preventive Intervention for Rural Low-Income African-American Pregnant Women at Risk for Postpartum Depression," *Archives of Women's Mental Health* 11, no. 5–6 (2008).

79. Crockett, "A Depression Preventive Intervention."

4. PAYING FOR TREATMENT

1. Carmen DeNavas-Walt, Bernadette D. Proctor, and Jessica C. Smith, U.S. Census Bureau, Current Population Reports, P60-245, *Income, Poverty, and Health Insurance Coverage in the United States: 2012*. Washington, DC: U.S. Government Printing Office, 2013.

2. DeNavas-Walt, *Income, Poverty, and Health Insurance Coverage in the United States: 2011*.

3. Kenneth Yeager et al., *Modern Community Mental Health: An Interdisciplinary Approach* (New York: Oxford University Press, 2013).

4. Yeager et al., *Modern Community Mental Health*.

5. DeNavas-Walt, *Income, Poverty, and Health Insurance Coverage in the United States: 2011*.

6. Gary Claxton et al., "Health Benefits in 2014: Stability in Premiums and Coverage for Employer-Sponsored Plans," *Health Affairs* 33, no. 10 (2014).

7. Claxton et al., "Health Benefits in 2014."

8. Claxton et al., "Health Benefits in 2014."

9. Leiyu Shi and Douglas A. Singh, *Essentials of the U.S. Health Care System* (Burlington, MA: Jones Bartlett, 2010).

10. U.S. Department of Defense, Tricare, http://www.tricare.mil.

11. U.S. Department of Defense, Tricare.

12. Catherine Hoffman and A. Schlobohm, *The Kaiser Commission on Medicaid and the Uninsured: Chart Book*, 2nd ed. (Washington, DC: Henry J. Kaiser Foundation, 2000).

13. Julia Paradise and Rachel Garfield, "What Is Medicaid's Impact on Access to Care, Health Outcomes, and Quality of Care? Setting the Record Straight on the Evidence," *Kaiser Commission on Medicaid and the Uninsured*, August (2013), http://kff.org/report-section/what-is-medicaids-impact-on-access-to-care-health-outcomes-and-quality-of-care-setting-the-record-straight-on-the-evidence-issue-brief/.

14. U.S. House of Representatives, House Committee on Ways and Means, "Green Book" (Washington, DC: GPO, 2012).

15. Centers for Medicare and Medicaid Services, "Medicare," http://www.cms.gov/Medicare/Medicare.html.

16. "Children's Health Insurance Program," http://www.medicaid.gov/chip/chip-program-information.html.

17. "The Mental Health Parity and Addiction Equity Act," http://www.cms.gov/CCIIO/Programs-and-Initiatives/Other-Insurance-Protections/mhpaea_factsheet.html.

18. "The Mental Health Parity and Addiction Equity Act."

19. John Holahan and Alshadye Yemane, "Enrollment Is Driving Medicaid Costs—but Two Targets Can Yield Savings," *Health Affairs* 28, no. 5 (2009).

20. Centers for Medicare and Medicaid Services, "Medicare."

21. Ian H. Gotlib and Constance L. Hammen, *Handbook of Depression*, third edition (New York: Guilford Press, 2014).

22. Mary Ellen O'Connell, Thomas Boat, and Kenneth E. Warner, National Research Council and Institute of Medicine, *Preventing Mental, Emotional, and Behavioral Disorders among Young People: Progress and Possibilities* (Washington, DC: National Academies Press, 2009).

Index